THE BEST MIND DIET COOKBOOK 2023

Guide For Alzheimer's And Brain Health

By

Ruth Luke

D1716051

Table of contents

Chapter one
Minds diet recipes for brain health

Chapter two
30 Smoothes and breakfast

Chapter three

12 best Salad soup and side

Chapter four

29 Fish and sea food

Introduction

MIND diet is a combination of the DASH diet and the Mediterranean diet that focuses on brain health specifically.

Everything you need to know about the MIND diet and how to follow it can be found in this comprehensive beginner's guide.

Mediterranean-DASH Intervention for Neurodegenerative Delay is the acronym for the MIND diet.

The MIND diet aims to prevent dementia and the deterioration of brain health that comes with age. It combines elements of the Mediterranean diet and the Dietary Approaches to Stop Hypertension p(DASH) diet, two very popular diets.

The Mediterranean and DASH diets are regarded as two of the healthiest by many experts. The MIND diet is a dietary pattern that combines the Mediterranean diet and the DASH diet to create a dietary pattern that focuses specifically on brain health. Research has shown that they can lower blood pressure and reduce the risk of heart disease, diabetes, and several other diseases.

Everything you need to know about the MIND diet and how to follow it can be found in this comprehensive beginner's guide.

The MIND diet:
"Mediterranean-DASH Intervention for Neurodegenerative Delay" is the acronym for "MIND."

The MIND diet aims to prevent dementia and the deterioration of brain health that comes with age. It combines elements of the Mediterranean diet and the Dietary Approaches to Stop Hypertension (DASH) diet, two very popular diets.

The Mediterranean and DASH diets are regarded as two of the healthiest by many experts. They have been shown in studies to lower blood pressure and lower the risk of diabetes, heart disease, and a number of other diseases.

However, the researchers wanted to develop a diet that would specifically assist in enhancing brain function and preventing dementia.

They did this by incorporating foods from the DASH and Mediterranean diets that had been shown to improve brain health.

The Mediterranean and DASH diets, for instance, both recommend consuming a lot of fruit. Berry consumption has been linked to improved brain function, whereas fruit consumption has not.

As a result, the MIND diet emphasises berries but not fruit consumption as a whole.

At this time, there are no predetermined instructions for following the MIND diet. You simply have the option of eating more of the ten foods that the diet suggests you avoid and fewer of the five foods that it suggests you avoid.

The diet's best and worst foods are discussed in the following two sections.

To aid in the prevention or postponement of cognitive decline, the MIND diet encourages the consumption of some foods and discourages the consumption of others. It incorporates aspects of other diets to encourage healthy eating habits that may lower Alzheimer's disease risk.

Memory, learning, and thought processing difficulties are all examples of cognitive impairment. Even though a lot of people may think that this is a normal part of getting older, it isn't a givenTrusted Source. According to Trusted Source, Alzheimer's disease, which causes cognitive decline, was the sixth leading cause of death in the United States in 2021. As a result, maintaining brain health is crucial, which may require eating a well-balanced, nutritious diet.

The Mediterranean and Dietary Approaches to Stop Hypertension (DASH) diets have been combined into the MIND diet, which has shown promise for preventing cognitive decline. People who follow this diet plan can help prevent the onset of Alzheimer's disease and maintain brain health by making a few easy changes to their diet.

Grains, legumes, fruits, nuts, vegetables, and fish are the primary components of the traditional Mediterranean diet. People can also consume alcohol, eggs, dairy, and meat in small quantities. Fruit, vegetables, and low-fat dairy products are emphasised in the DASH diet. Whole grains, poultry, fish, and nuts are also acceptable, but saturated fats, red meat, and sugars should be avoided.

While attempting to avoid saturated fats and added sugars, the MIND diet combines these dietary patterns by encouraging the consumption of numerous plant-based foods in addition to fish and poultry. The majority of the diet's differences come from its emphasis on daily and weekly recommendations for particular food groups and foods.

For instance, it states that two or more servings of vegetables should be consumed each day, but that at least one serving should consist of leafy green vegetables.

Depending on whether a person follows the MIND diet strictly or moderately well, there is evidence that it can help lower the risk of Alzheimer's disease by approximately 53% or 35%. This diet may be a promising strategy for preventing or delaying cognitive decline, despite the fact that additional research is required to confirm these findings. However, it is best to consult a physician before making any dietary changes.

The MIND diet aims to improve brain function and contribute to cognitive resilience in older adults, according to trusted sources. There is evidence to suggest that factors like a high-quality diet and a healthy lifestyle can benefit brain healthTrusted Source. As a result, following this diet may help slow cognitive decline and lower the risk of dementia and Alzheimer's disease.The MIND diet may also be linked to a slower rate of cognitive decline following a stroke, according to additional evidence.

Chapter one
Minds diet recipes for brain health

Benefits There is evidence to suggest that the MIND diet may have a number of advantages for a variety of people. It may also help prevent cardiovascular disease and some types of cancer, in addition to lowering the risk of Alzheimer's disease.

The risk of developing Alzheimer's disease may be increased by numerous factors. While some risk factors, such as age and genetics, cannot be changed, others, such as diet, cognitive training, and exercise, can be. According to the authors of a review published in 2019 by Trusted Source, the anti-inflammatory and antioxidant properties of some diets, such as the MIND diet, may assist in protecting the brain.

In a similar vein, the DASH dietTrusted Source and the Mediterranean dietTrusted Source both appear to have the potential to improve cardiovascular health. The MIND diet is probably also good for your heart because it combines elements of both diets.

Risks There are currently no known risks associated with the MIND diet. However, if a person wants to know if the diet is right for them, they should talk about it with a doctor.

Due to dietary preferences, allergies, or intolerances, some of the MIND diet's recommended foods may not be suitable for everyone. A person might want to talk to a doctor or dietitian about possible alternate diet plans in these situations.

green leafy vegetables, all other vegetables, berries, nuts, olive oil, whole grains, fish, beans, poultry, and wine are all included in the MIND diet's recommended daily intake. For instance, a person should aim to consume three or more servings of minimally processed whole grains per day and two or more servings of berries per week in addition to their daily intake of vegetables.

Avoidable foods The MIND diet also lists which foods to avoid. People should try to limit these foods as much as possible because it may not always be possible to do so.

less than one tablespoon of butter or margarine per day less than one serving of cheese per week less than four portions of red meat per week less than one serving of fast food or fried food items per week, on average, less than five servings of pastries and candies per week Meal plan example At this time, there are no established guidelines for adhering to the MIND diet. Instead, the goal is to encourage people to eat more of the ten recommended foods and fewer of the five that aren't as good for them. Therefore, a meal plan might include:

Oatmeal for breakfast is a practical choice. Oatmeal can be topped with fresh blueberries and walnuts to add vitamins and minerals, and it meets the MIND diet's requirements for whole grains.

Lunch: A pasta salad that can be made ahead of time is a good option for lunch. They can begin by adding spinach, tomato, cucumber, and chickpeas to a base of whole wheat pasta. To complete the meal, they can sprinkle salt and pepper on top and drizzle olive oil and balsamic vinegar over it.

Snacks Nuts can be a great on-the-go snack option. A person could also eat a piece of whole wheat bread spread with a thin layer of nut butter.

Dinner: Bake some lean chicken breast with fresh herbs and then coat it with a squeeze of fresh lemon for a filling and nutritious meal. They can serve it with quinoa and kale as a side. The MIND diet is an option for people who want to improve their cognitive health and overall brain function. The MIND diet, which stands for Mediterranean-DASH Intervention for Neurodegenerative Delay, combines two other healthy eating plans: The DASH eating plan, which was developed by the National Heart, Lung, and Blood Institute to assist in lowering blood pressure and enhancing heart health, is based on the eating habits of people who live in Mediterranean countries and has been shown to improve cardiovascular health.

The MIND diet combines elements of the two other diets with the intention of lowering the risk of cognitive decline and dementia, two conditions that frequently accompany ageing.According to Lisa Young, Ph.D., a registered dietitian nutritionist, adjunct professor of nutrition at New York University, and author of Finally Full, Finally Slim: A Diet to Prevent Cognitive Decline, "the premise is that you can reduce cognitive decline with a combination of the Mediterranean and DASH diets and by adding specific foods like leafy greens and berries." One portion at a time for 30 days to permanent weight loss.

Due to its emphasis on improving cognitive function, the MIND Diet is also distinct from the two diets from which it draws inspiration. With the exception of urging people to consume berries, it does not place as much emphasis on eating fish or fruit as the other options do. In addition, wine, which is not part of the DASH diet but is part of the Mediterranean diet, is included because moderate consumption has been linked to brain health[1].

1.Easy Fish Tacos with Kiwi Salsa These nutritious fish tacos can be made with cod or any firm white fish. The flavours and colours of the crispy tacos are enhanced by a vibrant kiwi salsa and red cabbage in this simple dinner recipe. Patience is the key to crispy, golden fish. Before adding the battered pieces, let the oil get hot. Before starting to cook, dip an instant-read thermometer into the oil to ensure that it is at the right temperature.

Ingredients: 1 cup sliced red cabbage, 1 tablespoon rice vinegar, 1 cup diced, peeled kiwi, 2 tablespoons finely diced red onion, 1 tablespoon chopped fresh cilantro, 1 tablespoon lime juice, 1 teaspoon finely chopped jalapeno pepper, plus slices for garnish, 1/4 cup divided white whole-wheat flour, 1 teaspoon baking powder, 1/4 teaspoon salt, plus a pinch, divided, 12 cups Mexican lager, 8 ounces skinned, centre-cut firm white In a small bowl, combine the kiwi, onion, cilantro, lime juice, and jalapeno. Place aside.

Step 2: In a medium bowl, whisk together beer, 1/2 cup flour, baking powder, and 1/4 teaspoon salt. Make eight pieces of fish. Use the remaining 1/4 cup of flour to dust. After shaking off any extra flour, add the fish to the batter and turn it over to coat.

Step 3: Arrange a wire rack on a baking sheet that is close to the stove. Heat oil in a medium skillet to 325 degrees Fahrenheit. Add half the fish to the pan and let the batter drip off. Cook for approximately three minutes, turning once, or until the coating is golden. Repeat with the remaining fish after moving them to a rack and allowing the oil to return to 325 degrees Fahrenheit. Add the remaining pinch of salt to the dish.

Step 4: If desired, top the fish with jalapeno slices, the reserved cabbage, and kiwi salsa.

2.Crispy Chickpea Grain Bowl with Lemon Vinaigrette

Our favourite component of these vegetarian grain bowls is the tangy lemon vinaigrette, which brings the quinoa, toasted pumpkin seeds, roasted chickpeas, kale, and quinoa together in a satisfying way. Make them for a healthy and filling dinner or easy lunches to prepare ahead of time.

Ingredients: 1/3 cup quinoa, 1 1/3 cups water, 1 tablespoon, divided; 1/8 teaspoon salt, 1/4 teaspoon, divided; 1 (15 ounce) can of no-salt-added chickpeas, rinsed; 1 small red onion, thinly sliced; 4 teaspoons extra-virgin olive oil, 2 tablespoons, divided; 1/4 teaspoon ground pepper, divided; 1 bunch kale, stems removed; thinly sliced (about 5 cups); 1 teaspoon Dijon mustard; 1

In a medium saucepan, combine the quinoa, 1/8 teaspoon salt, and 1 1/3 cups water. Over medium-high heat, bring to a boil. Reduce the heat to medium-low, partially cover, and simmer for about 15 minutes until the quinoa is tender. Get rid of any extra water.

Step 3: In the meantime, use a paper towel to dry the chickpeas. In a large bowl, toss with onion, 2 teaspoons of oil, and 1/8 teaspoon each of salt and pepper. Place on the baking sheet that has been prepared. Bake for fifteen minutes.

Step 4: In a large bowl, toss the kale with the remaining 1/8 teaspoon salt and 2 teaspoons of oil. After adding the kale to the chickpeas, roast for an additional 15 minutes.

Step 5: In a small bowl, combine the mustard, garlic, lemon juice, zest, remaining 1 tablespoon of water, and remaining 1/8 teaspoon of pepper. Add the remaining two tablespoons of oil with a whisk.

Step 6: Divide the quinoa among four bowls for serving. The kale mixture, bell pepper slices, feta, and pumpkin seeds should be served on top. Use the vinaigrette to drizzle.

3. Grilled Lemon-Pepper Salmon

in Foil We're willing to bet that this simple recipe for grilled salmon in foil will become a weekly dinner staple. Fish that has been cooked in foil stays extremely moist and does not stick to the grill. This adaptable main dish benefits from the addition of butter, fresh parsley, and lemon pepper. For a healthy dinner that is ready in less than 30 minutes, cook some vegetables alongside the fish packets, such as asparagus, zucchini, and corn.

Ingredients Checklist 4 skin-on salmon fillets (each 6 ounces) 2 tablespoons unsalted butter 1 teaspoon lemon pepper 12 teaspoon salt 8 thin slices of lemon (from 1 lemon) 4 sprigs of flat-leaf parsley Instructions Checklist Step 1 Preheat the grill to medium-high (400-450 degrees Fahrenheit). On a work surface, arrange four 12-inch-long foil squares in a single layer; spray cooking spray on. Place one salmon fillet in the middle of each, skin-side down. 1 1/2 teaspoons butter, 1/4 teaspoon lemon pepper, 1/8 teaspoon salt, 2 lemon slices, and 1 parsley sprig are the toppings for each fillet. To ensure a secure seal, crimp the sides of each foil packet together. On the grill, place the packets; Cover and grill for 8 to 10 minutes or until the fish flakes easily with a fork.

4. White Bean and Sun-Dried Tomato Gnocch

i Sun-dried tomatoes provide texture and umami in this dish. Ingredients: 12 cups sliced oil-packed sun-dried tomatoes, plus 2 tablespoons of oil from the jar, divided 1 package (16 ounces) shelf-stable gnocchi 1 can (15 ounces) low-sodium cannellini beans, rinsed 1 package (5 ounces) baby spinach 1 large shallot, minced 1 cup low-sodium no-chicken broth or chicken broth 1 cup heavy cream 1 tablespoon lemon juice 1 teaspoon salt 1 teaspoon ground pepper 3 tablespoons Gnocchi should be added and cooked for about 5 minutes, stirring frequently, until tender and beginning to brown.

Cook the beans and spinach for about one minute, or until the spinach is wilted. Place on a plate.

Step 2: Heat the pan over medium heat with the remaining 1 tablespoon of oil. Include shallot and sun-dried tomatoes; cook for one minute while stirring. Add broth as the heat goes up to high. Cook for about 2 minutes or until most of the liquid has evaporated.

Step 3: Stir in the cream, lemon juice, salt, and pepper after lowering the heat to medium. Mix the gnocchi mixture back into the pan to coat it in the sauce. Serve with basil on top.

5. Gnocchi with sun-dried tomato and white beans

This recipe's star ingredient is sun-dried tomatoes, which add texture and umami. Ingredients: 12 cup sliced oil-packed sun-dried tomatoes plus 2 tablespoons oil from the jar, divided 1 (16 ounce) package shelf-stable gnocchi 1 (15 ounce) can low-sodium cannellini beans, rinsed 1 (5 ounce) package baby spinach 1 large shallot, minced 13 cup low-sodium no-chicken broth or chicken broth 13 cup heavy cream 1 tablespoon lemon juice 14 teaspoon salt 14 teaspoon Gnocchi should be added and cooked for about 5 minutes, stirring frequently, until tender and beginning to brown. Cook the beans and spinach for about one minute, or until the spinach is wilted. Place on a plate.

Step 2: Heat the pan over medium heat with the remaining 1 tablespoon of oil. Include shallot and sun-dried tomatoes; cook for one minute while stirring. Add broth as the heat goes up to high. Cook for about 2 minutes or until most of the liquid has evaporated.

Step 3: Stir in the cream, lemon juice, salt, and pepper after lowering the heat to medium. Mix the gnocchi mixture back into the pan to coat it in the sauce. Serve with basil on top.

6. Crispy Tofu and Roasted Vegetable Grain Bowl with Pumpkin Seeds
This veggie-packed grain bowl inspired by burrito bowls is great for a quick and easy dinner or a packable lunch for work.

Ingredient List 8 ounces extra-firm tofu cut into 1-inch cubes; 5 tablespoons plus 1 teaspoon extra-virgin olive oil divided; 1 tablespoon reduced-sodium tamari or soy sauce (see Tip); 12 teaspoon chilli powder; 1 medium red bell pepper cut into 1/2-inch strips; 12 medium red onion cut into 1/2-inch wedges; 12 avocado; 13 cup water; 14 cup packed cilantro leaves, plus more for garnish;

Step 2: In a medium bowl, toss tofu, 1 tablespoon oil, chilli powder, and tamari (or soy sauce). Place on one side of the baking sheet that has been prepared. In a bowl, combine the pepper, onion, and 1 teaspoon of oil; toss to combine. On the opposite side of the baking sheet, arrange the vegetables. Roast for about 20 minutes, or until the tofu is hot and the vegetables are tender.

Step 3: In the meantime, in a blender jar or mini food processor, combine the remaining 4 tablespoons of oil, avocado, water, cilantro, lime juice, coriander, and salt. Scrape down the sides as necessary during processing until smooth.

Step 4: Divide 1/2 cup of the rice between two shallow serving bowls. Add the roasted vegetables, tofu, lettuce, and tomatoes on top. Sprinkle pumpkin seeds over each bowl with four tablespoons of dressing.

Tips and Advice: Because soy sauce may contain wheat or other flavors or sweeteners that contain gluten, people who have celiac disease or are sensitive to gluten should only use soy sauces that are marked "gluten-free."

7. Roasted Salmon Rice Bowl with Beets and Brussels

When you roast the salmon and vegetables together on a single sheet pan while the rice cooks, you get a simple and filling meal that is also full of whole grains, vegetables, and protein. Look for a wild rice blend that combines wild and brown rice to ensure that you are getting only whole grains.

Ingredient List 1 cup of wild rice blend 2 medium golden beets peeled and cut into 1/2-inch wedges 8 ounces trimmed and halved Brussels sprouts 3 tablespoons extra-virgin olive oil divided 3/4 teaspoon salt divided 3/4 teaspoon ground pepper divided 1 lemon 1 pound wild-caught salmon fillet divided into 4 portions 2 rosemary sprigs cut in half

2 tablespoons chopped fresh herbs such as thyme, basil, or rosemary 1 clove garlic minced 1 tablespoon chopped

Step 3: In a medium bowl, toss the beets and Brussels sprouts with 1 tablespoon of oil and 1/4 teaspoon each of salt and pepper. Spread the vegetables out on a large baking sheet with a rim and roast for about 15 minutes, or until just beginning to brown and soften, after the rice has cooked for 10 minutes.

Step 4: Split a lemon in half horizontally. Make four slices from one half of the lemon; reserve the other half. Place the salmon on the half of the baking sheet that is empty and move the Brussels sprouts and beets to one side. Add 1/4 teaspoon each of salt and pepper to the salmon, and garnish each piece with a rosemary sprig and a lemon slice. Continue roasting for another 9 to 11 minutes, or until the salmon is opaque in the middle and the vegetables have softened.

Step 5: In the meantime, put the juice from the remaining lemon half in a small bowl by squeezing it. Incorporate the herbs, garlic, and the remaining

1/4 teaspoon of salt and pepper with the remaining 2 tablespoons of oil.

Step 6: Split the rice into four bowls. Throw away the rosemary sprig and lemon slices. Place the vegetables and salmon on top of the rice. Sprinkle pistachios over each serving and drizzle with about 1 tablespoon of the mixture of lemon juice.

8. Herby Mediterranean Fish with Wilted Greens and Mushrooms

This recipe for Mediterranean fish is delicious and good for you on a weeknight. Serve with roasted potatoes or wild rice.

Ingredient List: 3 tablespoons olive oil, divided; 12 large sweet onions, sliced; 3 cups cremini mushrooms, sliced; 2 cloves garlic, sliced; 4 cups chopped kale, chopped; 1 medium tomato, diced; 2 teaspoons Mediterranean Herb Mix, divided; 1 tablespoon lemon juice, divided; 12 teaspoons salt, divided; 12 teaspoons ground pepper, divided; 4 (4 ounce) cod, sole, or tilapia fillets, divided; Chopped fresh parsley, for oil in a large, medium-sized saucepan. Add onion; cook, stirring occasionally, for three to four minutes until translucent. Add garlic and mushrooms; Cook, occasionally stirring, for 4 to 6 minutes or until the mushrooms begin to brown and release their liquid. Tomato, kale, and 1 tsp. herb blend. 5 to 7 minutes, or until the mushrooms are tender and the kale is wilted, stirring occasionally. Include 1/4 teaspoon and lemon juice. each pepper and salt Cover, remove from the heat, and remain warm.

Step 2: Sprinkle the remaining 1 teaspoon over the fish. 1/4 teaspoon of herb mixture each pepper and salt Heat the other two tablespoons. over medium-high heat, add oil to a large nonstick skillet. Cook the fish for 2 to 4 minutes per side, or until the flesh is opaque, depending on the thickness. The fish should be placed on four plates or a serving platter. Place the vegetables around the fish and top it; If desired, sprinkle with parsley.

9.Pickled Beet, Arugula, and Herbed Goat Cheese Sandwich

This sandwich of pickled beets, arugula, and goat cheese has a peppery flavour due to the creamy goat cheese and the sweet and tangy pickled beets. This simple sandwich gets its nuttiness and crunch from chopped walnuts.

Ingredients Ingredient Checklist 2 ounces softened goat cheese 1 tablespoon chopped fresh dill, 1 tablespoon snipped chives 1 teaspoon extra-virgin olive oil 1 teaspoon salt and pepper to taste 2 slices whole-wheat sandwich bread lightly toasted 1 tablespoon chopped walnuts, toasted 2 ounces sliced pickled beets 1 cup arugula Directions Instructions Checklist Step 1 Mash the goat cheese, chives, and dill together in a small bowl On one side of each piece of toast, spread the goat cheese mixture. Layer beets and arugula on top of one slice, then sprinkle with walnuts. Divide the sandwich in half and top with the second slice of toast, cheese-side down.

10.20-Minute Creamy Tomato Salmon Skillet

The salmon fillets cook quickly and are coated in a scrumptious, creamy sauce made with zucchini, tomatoes, and Italian seasoning. This simple salmon dinner is sure to become a new family favourite for weeknights. The good news is: This meal can be prepared in just 20 minutes.

Ingredients Ingredient Checklist 1 14 pounds of skinned salmon fillet, divided into four portions 14 teaspoon salt, divided 14 teaspoon ground pepper, divided 2 tablespoons olive oil, divided 1 medium zucchini, halved lengthwise and thinly sliced 12 cup chopped onion 13 cup dry white wine 1 (15 ounce) can of diced tomatoes without salt added 2 ounces cream cheese, cut into cubes 1 teaspoon Italian seasoning 12 teaspoon garlic powder 14 In a large skillet, heat 1 tablespoon of oil to medium-high heat. Cook the salmon for three to four minutes, or until the underside is browned and easily comes off the pan. Cook the salmon on the other side for another 2 to 3 minutes, or until opaque in the middle. Place on a plate.

Step 2: In the meantime, add the zucchini, onion, and the remaining 1 tablespoon of oil to the pan. Cook, stirring, for about three minutes until the vegetables begin to soften. Add the wine and raise the heat to medium-high. Cook, stirring, for about 2 minutes or until most of the liquid has evaporated. The remaining 1/8 teaspoon each of salt and pepper, tomatoes, cream cheese, Italian seasoning, and garlic powder are to be added. Stir constantly for 4 to 5 minutes or until the cream cheese is melted. Bring to a simmer. Turn the salmon over to coat it in the sauce after returning to the pan. Serve with basil on top.

11.Easy Tuna Cakes with Greens and Lemon Dressing

These easy tuna cakes over greens are made with canned tuna, white beans, and dried herbs. They are served with greens. This quick dinner is put together by a lemony dressing.

Ingredients: 12 cup rinsed, no-salt-added canned white beans 1 large egg lightly beaten 3 teaspoons divided Dijon mustard 1 teaspoon lemon zest 1 teaspoon dried dill 1 teaspoon dried mint 1 teaspoon dried tarragon 2 cans (5 ounces) wild albacore tuna packed in oil, drained 3/4 cup whole-wheat panko breadcrumbs 6 tablespoons extra-virgin olive oil, divided 3 tablespoons lemon juice 1 teaspoon honey 1 teaspoon ground pepper 1 Add the egg, 2 teaspoons of mustard, zest from the lemon, dill, mint, and tarragon. Slice the tuna into chunks; incorporate gently into the bean mixture. Sprinkle the mixture with panko; gently fold in until everything is well mixed. Make four patties from the mixture, each one-inch thick.

Step 2: In a large nonstick skillet, heat 1 tablespoon of oil over medium heat. To coat the pan, swirl. About three minutes per side, cook the patties until golden brown on both sides.

Step 3: In a small bowl, combine the honey, pepper, salt, lemon juice, remaining 1 teaspoon of mustard, and 5 tablespoons of oil. Divide the greens between four plates; Each with a tuna cake and dressing drizzled evenly on top.

12. Salmon with Walnut-Rosemary Crusted Walnuts and salmon are excellent sources of omega-3 fatty acids. Serve this straightforward salmon recipe with a straightforward salad and roasted potatoes or quinoa as a side.

Ingredients: Ingredient List 2 teaspoons Dijon mustard, 1 minced clove of garlic, 1 teaspoon lemon zest, 1 teaspoon lemon juice, 1 teaspoon chopped fresh rosemary, 1 teaspoon honey, 1 teaspoon kosher salt, 1 teaspoon crushed red pepper, 3 tablespoons panko breadcrumbs, 3 tablespoons finely chopped walnuts, 1 teaspoon extra-virgin olive oil, 1 pound skinless salmon fillet, fresh or frozen, Olive oil cooking spray, chopped fresh parsley, and lemon wedges for garnish

Step 2: In a small bowl, combine mustard, garlic, lemon juice, rosemary, honey, salt, and crushed red pepper. In a different small bowl, combine panko, walnuts, and oil.

Step 3: Place the salmon on the baking sheet you prepared. Sprinkle the panko mixture over the fish and press to adhere the mustard mixture. Spray some cooking spray all over it.

Step 4: Bake for 8 to 12 minutes, depending on the thickness, or until the fish flakes easily with a fork.

Step 5: Serve with lemon wedges if desired and sprinkle with parsley.

13.Shakshuka—Eggs Poached in Spicy Tomato Sauce

Shakshuka is a meal packed with vegetables that features eggs cooked in a mixture of spices, tomatoes, onions, and peppers. In North Africa and the Middle East, it is frequently served for breakfast or lunch.

Ingredient List 2 tablespoons olive oil 2 cups chopped red sweet peppers, 2 cups chopped onion, 2 tablespoons no-salt-added tomato paste, 1 teaspoon smoked paprika, 2 teaspoons crushed red pepper, 3 cups chopped tomatoes, 1 teaspoon ground cumin, 1/4 teaspoon salt, 4 eggs, 2 cups plain low-fat Greek yogurt, and 2 whole-wheat pita bread rounds, halved crosswise and warmed Through crushed red pepper, add the remaining five ingredients. Stir frequently after 5 to 7 minutes, or until the onion is tender. Add the salt, cumin, and tomatoes. Bring to the boil; halt the heat. Ten minutes or until the tomatoes begin to break down, simmer.

Step 2: In the tomato mixture, make four indentations. Slip an egg into an indentation in a custard cup or small bowl. With the remaining three eggs, continue. Cover and simmer for 4 to 6 minutes, or until the yolks begin to thicken but are not hard and the whites are completely set.

Step 3: Drizzle yogurt over the top and garnish with parsley. With pita bread, serve.

14.Chicken Burrito Bowls

This diabetic-friendly chicken burrito bowl eliminates the carb-heavy tortilla wrap.

Ingredient List 12 cup quinoa that has been rinsed and drained, 12 teaspoon ground cumin, 12 teaspoon salt, 12 teaspoon black pepper, 2 8-ounce skinless, boneless chicken breast halves that have been halved horizontally, 1 tablespoon olive oil, 14 of an avocado that has been peeled, 14 cup finely snipped fresh cilantro, 2 tablespoons plain fat-free Greek yogurt, 12 teaspoon lime juice, 1 can of rinsed and drained reduced-sodium pinto beans (3/4 cup), shredded reduced-fat cheddar cheese (1 ounce), and

2 tablespoons roasted and salted pumpkin seeds (pepitas) Instructions and Checklist Step 1: Follow

the package instructions to cook quinoa with cumin and 1/4 teaspoon salt and pepper.

Step 2: In the meantime, season the chicken on both sides with the remaining 1/4 teaspoon of salt and pepper. Heat oil in a 10-inch nonstick skillet on medium. Include chicken; cook, turning once, for 6 to 8 minutes or until no longer pink. Take out and let sit for five minutes. Slice in strips.

Step 3: Blend the yogurt, avocado, cilantro, and lime juice in a small bowl until nearly smooth. Add milk to thin to a drizzling consistency if desired.

Step 4: Divide the lettuce among the bowls. Add chicken, quinoa, tomatoes, beans, avocado mixture, cheese, and pepitas to the top.

15. Cajun-Spiced Tofu Tostadas with Beet Crema
These tostadas have a juicy mango slaw on top of crumbled tofu that has been seasoned with Cajun seasoning. Even more flavor is added by mixing lime and beets into sour cream. In the produce

section of your grocery store, look for beets that have already been cooked.

Ingredients: 8 corn tortillas, 2 tablespoons avocado oil, divided, 3 cups shredded cabbage, 12 mango, julienned (see tip), 2 tablespoons lime juice, divided, 1 tablespoon chopped fresh cilantro, 4 teaspoon salt, divided, 1 small cooked beet, shredded, 13 cups sour cream, 1 small clove garlic, grated, 14 to 16 ounce package extra-firm tofu, drained, crumbled, and patted dry, 2 tablespoons salt-free Cajun heat to 400°F.

Step 2: Arrange the tortillas on a baking sheet and brush both sides with 1 tablespoon oil. It's okay if some of them overlap; As they cook, they will shrink.) Bake for 10 to 12 minutes, turning once halfway through, or until crisp and browned. Cool on a wire rack after transferring.

Step 3: In the meantime, combine cabbage, mango, cilantro, 1/4 teaspoon salt, and 1 tablespoon lime juice in a medium bowl. In a small bowl, combine the beet, sour cream, garlic, remaining lime juice, and 1/4 teaspoon salt.

Step 4: In a large cast-iron skillet, heat the remaining 1 tablespoon of oil to medium-high heat. Tofu, the remaining 1/4 teaspoon of salt, and Cajun seasoning. 8 to 10 minutes, stirring occasionally, or until nicely browned.

Step 5: Spread avocado, tofu, slaw, and beet crema on top of the tostadas.

16. Rice and Salmon Bowl

Lunch or dinner can be satisfied with this tasty bowl. You can have a filling and flavorful meal in just 25 minutes with a few healthy ingredients like instant brown rice, heart-healthy salmon, and a lot of crunchy vegetables. Do you want to cut back on carbs? Try substituting riced cauliflower for brown rice.

Ingredients Checklist 4 ounces of salmon, preferably wild, 1 teaspoon avocado oil 1/8 teaspoon kosher salt 1 cup instant brown rice 1 cup water 2 tablespoons mayonnaise 1/12 teaspoon Sriracha 1/12 teaspoon 50%-less-sodium tamari 1/12 teaspoon mirin 1/12 teaspoon freshly grated ginger 1/4 teaspoon crushed red pepper 1/8 teaspoon kosher salt 12 sheets nori (roasted seaweed) Directions Checklist Step 1 Preheat the oven to 400 degrees Fahrenheit. Line Salmon should be placed on the prepared pan. Apply oil to it; Add salt to taste. Bake for 8 to 10 minutes, or until an instant-read thermometer inserted into the thickest part registers 125°F.

Step 2: In the meantime, in a small saucepan, combine the rice and water; Follow the package's instructions to cook. In a small bowl, combine Sriracha and mayonnaise; place aside. In a separate small bowl, combine the tamari, mirin, ginger, crushed red pepper, and salt; place aside.

Third step: Divide the rice into two bowls. Add salmon, avocado, cucumber, and kimchi to the top. Apply the mayonnaise and tamari mixtures as a drizzle. If desired, combine the bowls and serve with nori.

17. Roasted Maple-Glazed Chicken with Carrots

In a hot oven, olive oil and maple syrup turn into a sticky, sweet sauce. The flavor of the carrots is enhanced even further by drizzling the chicken drippings over them.

Ingredient List: 1 tablespoon finely chopped fresh rosemary, 2 sprigs, divided; 34 teaspoon salt, divided; 14 teaspoon ground pepper; 4 bone-in, skin-on chicken thighs (approximately 1 3/4 pounds each); 1 pound medium carrots, halved lengthwise if large; 2 tablespoons extra-virgin olive oil; 2 tablespoons pure maple syrup heat to 450°F.

Step 2: In a small bowl, combine chopped rosemary, 1/2 teaspoon salt, and pepper. Apply the mixture to the chicken's skin and any meat that is still visible. On a large baking sheet with a rim, place the chicken skin side up. On yet another large baking sheet with a rim, arrange the carrots in an even layer.

Step 3: In a small bowl, combine the oil and maple syrup. Apply the brush to the carrots and chicken. Add rosemary sprigs to the pan and sprinkle the carrots with the remaining 1/4 teaspoon of salt.

Step 4: Roast the chicken for 20 to 25 minutes on the upper rack until golden and 165°F on an instant-read thermometer inserted into the thickest part without touching the bone. Roast the carrots simultaneously on the lower rack for 20 to 25 minutes, stirring once, until tender and caramelized. Toss the carrots with the chicken drippings to coat. The carrots should accompany the chicken.

18.Sheet-Pan Shrimp and Beets
The beets get a head start in the oven for this simple dinner on a sheet pan while you prepare the shrimp and kale. Leave the shrimp tails intact for a more attractive presentation. A refreshing glass of rosé goes well with this one-pan recipe.

Ingredients Checklist 1 pound small beets, peeled and cut into 1/2-inch pieces 2 tablespoons extra-virgin olive oil, divided 34 teaspoon salt, divided 34 teaspoon ground pepper, divided 6 cups chopped kale 1 14 pounds extra-large raw shrimp, deveined and peeled 12 teaspoons dry mustard 12 teaspoons dried tarragon 3 tablespoons unsalted sunflower seeds, toasted Instructions Checklist Step 1 Preheat oven to 425 degrees F On a baking sheet with a rim, distribute evenly. Bake for fifteen minutes.

Step 3: In a bowl, toss the kale with the remaining oil, 1/4 teaspoon each of salt and pepper. Blend in with the beets that are on the baking sheet.

Step 4: Toss the shrimp with the remaining 1/4 teaspoon each of salt and pepper, mustard, and tarragon. Spread over the vegetables. Roast for an additional 10 to 15 minutes, or until the shrimp are cooked and the vegetables are tender.

Step 5: Arrange the shrimp on a platter for serving. Serve the vegetables with the shrimp and incorporate the sunflower seeds.

19. Baked Fish Tacos with Avocado This five-ingredient recipe for quick and easy fish tacos uses baked fish fillets instead of deep-frying them. These tacos can be made with a variety of flaky white fish. The best way to buy fish at the market is to be flexible and select the variety that looks the freshest that day.

Ingredients Checklist 1 tablespoon avocado oil 2 teaspoons no-salt-added Mexican-style seasoning blend 2 teaspoons salt 1 pound flaky white fish fillets, such as cod, haddock, or mahi mahi, cut into 8 or 16 pieces 1 avocado cut into 16 slices 12 cup pico de gallo 8 warmed corn tortillas Instructions Checklist Step 1 Coat a large baking sheet with cooking spray.

Step 2: In a medium bowl, combine the salt, seasoning mix, and oil. Toss in the fish to coat. Place the fish on the baking sheet that has been prepared, and bake for 10 to 15 minutes, depending on the thickness.

Step 3: Place one or two fish pieces, two avocado slices, and one tablespoon pico de gallo in each tortilla to make tacos.

20.Vegetarian Chopped Power Salad with a Creamy Cilantro Dressing When blended into a creamy dressing, cilantro adds color and flavor. This nutritious salad can be served for lunch or dinner.

Ingredients Ingredient Checklist 12 cup chopped cilantro 14 cup buttermilk 14 cup mayonnaise 2 tablespoons chopped shallot 1 tablespoon cider vinegar 14 teaspoon salt 14 teaspoon ground pepper 6 cups torn lettuce 2 cups finely sliced stemmed kale 1 (15 ounce) can rinsed chickpeas 2 medium carrots 1 medium red or yellow bell pepper, diced 1 cup cooked quinoa 13 cup roasted unsalted pepitas Directions Instructions Blend well with the processor.

Step 2: In a large bowl, combine quinoa, bell pepper, kale, chickpeas, carrots, and lettuce. Sprinkle the salad with the dressing and toss it well to coat. Before serving, sprinkle with pepitas.

21.Pumpkin Seed Salmon with Maple-Spice Carrots

This one-pan meal is ready in 35 minutes, making it a good choice for a healthy recipe after a long day at work. Pepita-crusted salmon fillets and maple-spiced carrots cook together to make a meal that everyone in the family will love.

Ingredients Checklist 4 fresh or frozen salmon fillets (4-5 ounces) 1 pound carrots (cut diagonally into 1/4-inch slices) 1 cup pure maple syrup (divided) 12 teaspoons salt (divided) 12 teaspoons pumpkin pie spice (divided) 8 multi-grain saltine crackers (finely crushed) 3 tablespoons finely chopped salted, roasted pumpkin seeds (pepitas) plus 2 teaspoons, divided Cooking spray Line a 15x10-inch baking pan with foil and preheat the oven to 425 degrees F. place aside.

Step 2: In a large bowl, combine the pumpkin pie spice, carrots, three tablespoons of maple syrup, and one-fourth teaspoon of salt. On one half of the prepared baking pan, arrange the carrots. For ten minutes, bake.

Step 3: Rinse the fish in the interim; With paper towels, wipe dry. In a shallow dish, combine crushed crackers, three tablespoons of pumpkin seeds, and the remaining 1/4 teaspoon salt. Apply the remaining 1 tablespoon of maple syrup to the fish's top. Press the cracker mixture into the surface to adhere. The fish should be placed in the baking pan alongside the carrots. Spray cooking spray all over the fish's top. Bake an additional 10 to 15 minutes, or until the carrots are tender and the fish flakes easily with a fork.

Step 4: Distribute the carrots on dinner plates and sprinkle them with the remaining 2 teaspoons of pumpkin seeds before serving. Add the salmon on top.

Chapter two
30 Smoothes and breakfast

We have to agree that smoothies are now a go-to meal option for health-conscious individuals: They're packed with fruits and vegetables, easy to make, and ready in a flash. However, not every smoothie is created equal. In fact, many store-bought smoothies contain a lot of calories and sugar. Therefore, if you are looking for healthy smoothie recipes, we have the ingredients and expert-approved techniques that you should immediately throw into your blender.

How to make a healthy smoothie Smoothies can be a healthy breakfast option if they contain the right amount of protein, carbohydrates, and healthy fats.

She adds that adding vegetables, flax seeds, hemp seeds, or chia seeds, a source of healthy fat like nuts or avocado, and additional fiber like flax, hemp, or chia seeds can also help provide essential vitamins, minerals, and antioxidants.

Is drinking a smoothie every day healthy?

If you want to start making smoothies at home with your own blender, you are already one step ahead of the game in terms of saving money and ensuring that you have complete control over the ingredients. It's fine to drink a smoothie every day as long as the nutrients are balanced well.

However, according to dietitians, chewing and swallowing food is actually preferable to drinking it to feel full, so you should probably stick to one smoothie per day and eat regular meals and snacks throughout the day. Additionally, try to include at least 25 grams of protein in your smoothie if you want to turn it into a meal. If it's a snack, aim for 10 grams of protein or more.

With nutrient-dense fruits and vegetables, creamy milk, protein, probiotic-rich yogurt, and other healthy ingredients, these delicious smoothies make healthy eating simpler. A quick note: For added sweetness, some of these recipes use honey or fruit juice, but if you want to avoid added sugar, you can eliminate those ingredients.

1. Blueberry Smoothie Bowl

Is it true that smoothies are only meant to be sipped? Almond milk, almond butter, and frozen blueberries can all be combined in a blender to create a delectable, ultra-creamy dessert. For the breakfast bowl of your dreams, decorate with fresh blueberries, hemp seeds, vanilla granola, and more after dividing into two bowls.

Ingredients: 1 cup frozen blueberries, 1/2 cup unsweetened almond milk, 1.5 scoops protein powder, and 2 tablespoons 1 teaspoon unsweetened almond butter 1/2 cup fresh blueberries, 1/4 cup vanilla granola, and 2 tablespoons pure vanilla extract 2 teaspoons sliced almonds 1 teaspoon hemp seeds Step 1: Puree frozen blueberries, almond milk, protein powder, almond butter, and vanilla in a blender until smooth. Split into two bowls.
Step 2: Before serving, top each bowl with cinnamon, fresh blueberries, granola, almonds, and hemp seeds.

2. Berry, Chia, and Mint Smoothie
This ruby smoothie with strawberries, raspberries, and beets is our favorite color. You'll get a lot of

gut-friendly fiber from it, and the unexpected addition of mint will make it refreshing.

Ingredients: 1/3 cup mint leaves, 1/2 cup sliced strawberries, 1/2 cup grated beet (from a medium beet), and 1 tbsp. chia seeds 1 cup unsweetened almond milk Instructions: Step 1: Place the berries, beets, mint, and chia seeds in a freezer-safe jar or plastic bag that can be resealed. Freeze for at least an hour.

Step 2: When you're ready to start, add frozen ingredients and almond milk to the blender. Blend until it is smooth. Use two tall glasses to serve.

3.Green Pineapple Coconut Smoothie

Baby spinach adds a nutritional punch to the tropical flavors of pineapple, coconut, banana, and lime. It's a healthy cup that will make you feel like you're on an island vacation at any time of day.

2 cups baby spinach, 1 cup frozen pineapple chunks, 1 cup light coconut milk, 1 frozen sliced banana, and 1 teaspoon 1 tablespoon grated lime zest Instructions for lime juice In a blender, blend all ingredients until smooth. Split into two glasses.

4.Stress Less Smoothie Tangy kefir has benefits for the gut and, when paired with raspberries, hemp seeds, and a peach, it might help you feel less stressed. But if you can't find hemp seeds, you can get a similar boost of magnesium, which is important for reducing stress, by adding a tablespoon of almond butter.

5.Creamy Kale Smoothie

This smoothie is from Prevention's Smoothies & Juices section titled "Balanced Gut." Greek yogurt is a natural supplement for gut health that is loaded with protein and probiotics.

Blend 1/2 cup plain Greek yogurt, 1/2 cup unsweetened almond milk, 1 teaspoon honey, and 1 cup coarsely chopped kale in a blender.

6.Citrus-Pineapple Smoothie Bowl

This smoothie bowl is a fun way to change up your routine. Blend until the mixture is smooth and frothy. It includes citrus fruits high in vitamin C, cashews that are good for the heart, and Greek yogurt that is good for the gut.

In a blender, combine half a cup of fat-free Greek yogurt, half a cup of frozen pineapple chunks, one teaspoon of vanilla extract, one navel orange segmented, and one ruby grapefruit segmented. Divide the mixture between two bowls and blend until smooth. Add chia seeds, chopped cashews, unsweetened coconut flakes, and additional orange and grapefruit to the top.

7.Peach Blueberry Smoothie

This sweet combination of blueberries and peaches will make you feel like it's summer even though it's winter. Kale is full of nutrients, so you'll get your daily dose of greens from it. Cinnamon is the perfect finishing touch.

Blend 1 cup chilled almond or vanilla soy milk, four peach slices (about 1/2 cup), 1/4 cup blueberries, a handful of kale, and 1/4 teaspoon in a blender. granulated cinnamon Blend until it is smooth.

8. Banana-Blueberry-Soy Smoothie This healthy smoothie is loaded with potassium-rich banana and vanilla for sweetness. The succulent blueberries in it are bursting with flavor.

Simply combine one teaspoon of pure vanilla extract, one cup of frozen blueberries, one frozen banana, and one cup of light soy milk. Blend until smooth, about 20 to 30 seconds. If you'd like the mixture to be thinner, you can add up to 1/4 cup more milk.

9.Peaches and Cream Oatmeal Smoothie
 Don't have time for a leisurely meal? Try this quick and easy version of morning oatmeal that is loaded with probiotics. Prebiotic fiber in whole-grain oats aids in gut health.

Two smoothies are made with this recipe from Prevention's Smoothies & Juices: Blend 1 cup frozen peaches, 1 cup frozen banana, 1/2 cup ice,

1/2 cup rolled oats, and 1/2 cup whole milk until smooth.

10. Pineapple Passion Smoothie

Your desire for an ice cream cone will be satisfied by this decadently thick smoothie recipe. Additionally, bromelain, an enzyme that aids in the breakdown of protein and may reduce bloating, is found in pineapple.

Six ice cubes, one cup of pineapple chunks, and one cup of low-fat or light vanilla yogurt should be combined.

11.Milk and Honey Smoothie

Make use of the celery in your produce drawer with this blended juice, which combines it with almond milk, cucumber, and grapes for a snack worthy of a sip. Pulse as necessary to achieve a smooth mixture.

Blend 1 1/2 cups unsweetened almond milk, 1 medium Kirby cucumber, 1 cup seedless green grapes, 2 medium stalks celery, and 1 tablespoon honey in a blender. Serves 2 and is blended until smooth.

12.Silky Skin Smoothie

This Smoothies and Juices from Prevention drink is great for your skin! The antioxidant beta-carotene, which the body converts into vitamin A, is abundant in apricots and carrots. This vitamin may protect the skin from damage caused by pollution and ultraviolet rays as well as from aging.

Blend 1/2 cup ice cubes, 1/2 cup Greek yogurt made with whole milk, 1/4 cup grated carrot, 1/2 teaspoon cinnamon, 2 chopped dried apricots, and 1 chopped fresh apricot (pitted and coarsely chopped) in a blender. Blend until it is smooth.

13.Lean, Mean, Green Machine

This smoothie is perfect for a post-workout recovery drink. Protein powder helps you get the energy you burn back, sweet bananas, kiwis, and coconut water give you potassium and vitamin C, and coconut water rehydrates you.

Add one medium banana that has been cut into pieces, one kiwi that has been peeled and cut into pieces, one cup of spinach, one scoop of vanilla whey protein powder, and half a cup of coconut water to a blender. Pulse until smooth and creamy.

14. Berry-Banana-Oat Smoothie

Oats give smoothies more body, and the resistant starch in this whole grain makes you feel fuller for longer. Is resistant starch also beneficial? Compared to other fibers, it produces less gas.

Blend 1 cup vanilla low-fat yogurt, 2 cups frozen strawberries, 1 sliced banana, 1/2 cup rolled oats, 1/2 cup orange juice, and 1 teaspoon honey in a blender. Serve 4 after blending the mixture until smooth.

15. Caribbean Dream Smoothie

If you often feel uneasy in your stomach before big events, you might want to drink this smoothie from Prevention's Smoothies & Juices. It includes banana, which contains magnesium, a calming mineral; Additionally, the probiotics in the yogurt may reduce anxiety.

Blend 1/4 cup refrigerated unsweetened coconut milk, 1/4 cup orange juice, 1/4 large banana, 1/2 cup pineapple chunks, and a handful of ice cubes until smooth. Take it two hours before you need to calm down for the best results in reducing anxiety.

16.Green Ginger Smoothie

The refreshing green color of this smoothie is the result of the combination of baby spinach and Granny Smith apples. Healthy fats and plant protein are added by hemp seeds.

Combine 2 cups packed baby spinach, 1 granny smith apple chopped, 3/4 cup coconut water, 1/4 cup lemon juice, and 2 tablespoons. 3 tsp. hemp seeds 1 tsp. minced ginger 1 1/2 cups ice and raw honey Blend until it is smooth. Serves two people.

17.Cranberry Banana Smoothie

The star of this satiating, fiber-rich dessert is the autumn berry. Almond milk reduces calories, bananas give the dish body and sweetness, and maple syrup provides a seasonal sweetness.

Blend 1 banana, 1 cup unsweetened almond milk, 1 cup frozen cranberries, and 1 teaspoon in a blender. ice cubes, 12 cups of maple syrup. Blend until smooth and frothy.

18.Apple Crisp Smoothie

This delicious smoothie is made with sweet apple cider, Greek yogurt, oats, nuts, and warming spices to bring out the flavors of fall. Additionally, it is high in beta-glucan, a type of fiber that boosts endurance, and protein.

Ingredients: 1 cup apple cider, 1/2 cup greek yogurt with 2% vanilla, 1/4 cup old-fashioned rolled oats, and 2 tablespoons. 1/4 teaspoon pecans cinnamon, 14 teaspoon nutmeg 1 cup ice cubes Instructions: Blend the ingredients and enjoy.

19.Green Tea, Blueberry, and Banana Smoothie

Simply heat three tablespoons of the antioxidant-rich green tea to make this smoothie. of water in a microwave-safe bowl until piping hot. After that, add one bag of green tea and let it brew for three minutes. Mix in 2 teaspoons after removing the tea bag. honey to dissolve it. In a blender, combine 3/4 cup calcium-fortified light vanilla soy milk, 1/2 medium banana, and 1 1/2 cups frozen blueberries. After adding the tea, process everything until smooth.

20.Mocha Protein Shake

This effervescent breakfast resembles a milkshake in flavor. What is the secret? Walnuts. Omega-3 fatty acids, which are known to help fight inflammation and protect your heart, and protein are abundant in these nuts. This is the ideal breakfast shake thanks to the addition of black coffee.

Blend 1 1/2 cups cooled black coffee, 1 large chunked frozen banana, 1 cup ice cubes, 1/4 cup walnuts, and 1 heaping teaspoon in a blender. 6 tablespoons of unsweetened cocoa powder powdered chocolate protein Blend until it is smooth. This recipe serves two.

21. Powerhouse Pumpkin Smoothie This smoothie contains Greek yogurt in addition to pure pumpkin for a creamy, protein-rich base. Seasonal sweetness is provided by pumpkin pie spice and maple syrup.

Combine 7 ounces and 1/2 cup of frozen canned pure pumpkin in a blender. 2 tablespoons, 1/4 avocado, and 1/2 cup water in 2% Greek yogurt 1 Tbsp ground flaxseed maple syrup and half a teaspoon spice for pumpkin pie. Blend till smooth.

22.Strawberry-Kiwi Smoothie

In a blender, combine 1 1/4 cup cold apple juice, 1 ripe banana, 1 kiwi, 5 frozen strawberries, and 1 1/2 teaspoon honey to make this fruity, low-calorie smoothie recipe even healthier. Organic kiwis contain more vitamin C and polyphenols that are good for the heart. Blend till smooth.

23. Tropical Papaya Perfection Smoothie

This breakfast smoothie with coconut added tastes just like a milkshake. You'll be transported to a tropical island with just one sip.

Blend one papaya with one cup of fat-free plain yogurt, half a cup of fresh pineapple chunks, half a cup of crushed ice, and one teaspoon. 1 tsp. coconut extract pulverized flaxseed The mixture should be processed for about 30 seconds, or until it is frosty and smooth.

24. Banana Almond Protein Smoothie

Creamy almond butter provides healthy fats, and coconut water assists in the replenishment of electrolytes following a strenuous workout. The high protein content is maintained by a scoop of whey and Greek yogurt.

Add 3 tablespoons, 1/2 cup plain Greek yogurt, and 1/2 cup coconut water to a blender. 1 tablespoon of almond butter, 1 scoop of whey protein powder 1 cup ice, hemp seeds, and a frozen banana Blend until smooth. This recipe makes enough for 2.

25.Berry Good Workout Smoothie

This simple smoothie recipe will give you the energy you need to power through your workout in just a few minutes. Try adding a teaspoon of Organic Kale Powder to your diet for an additional calcium boost.
You will need: 1/2 cup each of chopped strawberries, blueberries, and raspberries, and 2

tablespoons 1 teaspoon honey ice cubes, fresh lemon juice, and half a cup Blend until it is smooth.

26. Tutti-Frutti Smoothie

Citrus is infused into this healthy and refreshing snack with a splash of orange juice. You only need half a cup each of mixed frozen berries, half a cup each of plain yogurt, half a cup each of sliced ripe banana, and half a cup each of orange juice and canned crushed pineapple in juice. Approximately two minutes, or until smooth, process. Two people can eat this. Use fresh pineapple instead of canned pineapple and orange juice to reduce sugar.)

27. Mango Madness Smoothie

This delicious smoothie recipe makes use of the ability of ripe mangoes to fight disease. First, in a blender, combine one can of juice-packed pineapple chunks, one cup of fat-free frozen vanilla yogurt, one large mango that has been peeled and pitted, and one ripe banana. Blend until it is smooth. Then, add ice in small amounts, about 4 cups, until the mixture is pureed. A frothy, creamy drink that's perfect for two people comes out of this.

28. Antioxidant Berry Avocado Smoothie

This smoothie recipe uses frozen avocado for a super-creamy texture and is loaded with nutrients and antioxidants. In addition, the combination of frozen berries, spinach, flax seeds, and an antioxidant-rich blend add great flavor and fill you up.

Ingredients: 1 cup Sprouts Whole Antioxidant Blend, 1 cup Sprouts Sliced Frozen Avocados, 1 banana, 1 handful of spinach, 2 tablespoons ground flax seeds, and 1 cup unsweetened almond milk. Instructions: Place all ingredients in the blender and blend until smooth and creamy, then garnish with fresh berries.

If you want the consistency to be thinner, you can add more milk.

Fill a glass with your preferred toppings, such as fresh berries, and enjoy!

29. Caramel Apple Overnight Oatmeal Smoothie

This vegan, gluten-free breakfast smoothie is ideal for chilly mornings when you're in the mood for something sweet from the fall season. No worries: This recipe does not contain any caramel. Instead, this blogger substitutes dates for sugar to provide antioxidants, fiber, minerals, and natural sweetness. In addition to providing protein and fiber, rolled oats have the flavor of apples and cinnamon, which is undeniably comforting. You can save a lot of time in the morning by chilling this dreamy mixture overnight.

Ingredients: 12 cup (40 g) rolled oats**, 1 tbsp (7 g) chia seeds, 1/2 tsp ground cinnamon, 1 medium apple, peeled and cored (120 g), 2 pitted Medjool dates (30 g), 1 cup (240 ml) unsweetened vanilla almond milk*** Instructions: The night before, combine all of the ingredients in the bowl of your blender and give it a good stir to make sure Cover and refrigerate at least three hours, preferably overnight.

Blend the smoothie the next morning until it is smooth and creamy, adding more milk if it is too thick. Add the toppings you want and serve in a bowl or glass.

30. Carrot Cake Smoothie

Carrots aren't typically the star of a breakfast smoothie, but this luscious combination will convince you otherwise. This veggie-packed smoothie tastes exactly like a slice of carrot cake because the carrots go well with banana slices, diced pineapple, walnuts, cinnamon, and nutmeg, and it's packed with vegetables.

Carrots are the ingredients. Carrots are truly nature's candy, sweet but full of vitamin A, fiber, potassium, vitamin C, and manganese.
Pineapple. To keep the smoothie from getting too watery, I use frozen pineapple in place of ice.
Banana. makes the smoothie creamy and thicker.
Yogurt from Greece possesses the tang of a cream cheese frosting without the calories or fat.
Cashew Juice adds protein and unsaturated fats that are good for your heart while thinning the smoothie to a drinkable consistency.

Coconut. Feel free to leave out the coconut if you don't like it, but I love how it goes with the carrot, pineapple, banana, and cinnamon. Yum!

Nutmeg and cinnamon. Include the essential flavor of carrot cake in the recipe.

Walnuts. adds a hint of nuts to the smoothie and healthy omega-3 fats and antioxidants to this dessert that can be drunk.

The Instructions Blend all of the ingredients together.

Pour into a glass and garnish as desired after blending until silky smooth. ENJOY

Chapter three
12 best Salad soup and side

1. Balsamic Vinaigrette

Any home cook who wants to try their hand at salads will need a good vinaigrette. Fortunately, making delicious dressing is so simple. A winning dressing can be made by combining high-quality olive oil, vinegar, salt, pepper, and possibly a little honey in a jar. It will help elevate the flavor of your salads to new heights and can be stored for days in the refrigerator.

The fundamental proportion Three parts olive oil to one part vinegar is the fundamental ratio for any vinaigrette. Because the acidity of vinegars can vary greatly, this ratio is meant to be flexible.

Feel free to increase the amount of vinegar or decrease the amount of olive oil if you prefer a dressing that is more tart or if you have a vinegar with a milder flavor, such as white balsamic.

By extending this fundamental ratio, you can produce some truly amazing combinations.

You can try substituting a different kind of vinegar for the plain balsamic, or you can add new ingredients to change the entire dressing.

Consider the following flavor additions: For more ideas, see our Soups and Salads page).

Herby: Add one to two tablespoons of fresh or one to two teaspoons of dried herbs, such as dill, basil, or Italian, to the dish. Cheesy: Sprinkle Garlicky with 1 to 2 tablespoons grated Parmesan: Mustard-y: Add one to two teaspoons of finely minced garlic. How to make balsamic vinaigrette This recipe for balsamic vinaigrette only requires a few ingredients and can be made in a matter of seconds. You only need to combine everything and toss it in your salad—no need for a food processor or mixer!

The recipe is lovely if you want a sophisticated but not overpowering vinaigrette, and the few ingredients let all the flavors shine. Spend a little extra money on a bottle of high-quality, aged balsamic vinegar to get the best results. It will give this recipe more depth and complexity.

Additionally, you should try to use extra-virgin olive oil because it adds flavor without making the vinaigrette overly oily.

Salad with balsamic vinaigrette This recipe for balsamic vinaigrette is extremely adaptable and goes well with the majority of salads.

I'm going to show you two salad recipes that go well with this vinaigrette. You'll love the delicious flavours in both!

In a bowl, combine some mixed greens (such as Brussel sprouts, arugula, and spinach) with tomato slices and feta cheese cubes for the first recipe. Red onions, thinly sliced, can also be added for a kick. Add two tablespoons of the vinaigrette at the end and toss to combine.

The second recipe combines this tart vinaigrette with the delightful combination of apples and walnuts to provide you with the best of both worlds. Toss some lettuce, apple cubes, walnuts, feta, and vinaigrette in a bowl, then enjoy!

Alternately, you could use this dressing on our kale pomegranate salad.

Honey-balsamic vinaigrette This recipe for balsamic vinaigrette substitutes honey for sugar.

In addition to being healthier than sugar, honey has a milder flavor and provides the vinaigrette with delightful floral notes. If you don't want your vinaigrette to be too sweet, this is a great option!

You can easily make your vinaigrette at home using this recipe rather than purchasing a bottle from the store, which will probably cost a lot more. Anyone can make this recipe, and you can even modify it to suit your preferences.

You might be managing a family member's health, struggling to lose or maintain a healthy weight, or leading a busy life.

Your meals will be planned for you by our Meal Plan Membership. Enjoy your healthy meal plan and stop worrying about dinner.

You will receive substitution suggestions and shopping lists for the Mediterranean Diet each month. Our recipes don't use strange ingredients and are quick, simple, delicious, and healthy. You can save even more time by using leftovers in our meal plans!

2. Roasted Romaine Lettuce

Greens roasted in the oven sounds insane.

That is to say, before you try it, it sounds insane.

The lettuce appears to simply shrivel up or become mush. It is difficult to comprehend how the oven transforms a basic salad ingredient into a roasty, garlicky side dish that rivals any main dish.

However, if you've ever roasted other vegetables, you know that when olive oil, vegetables, and some heat are combined, something magical happens in the oven.

You may have noticed that roasting vegetables is one of our favourite pastimes around here!

How good are leafy greens for you?
You probably know how much we enjoy leafy green vegetables if you read this blog or other Mediterranean diet blogs.

First, greens contain a lot of fiber and very few calories. Second, all kinds of greens, including romaine, are high in folate, potassium, calcium, and vitamins C, A, K, and B.

Due to its high nutrition and low calorie content, romaine is referred to by Healthline as a "dieter's dream." We call it a dream for anyone who wants to live a healthy life because of all the essential vitamins and minerals in those leaves!

This recipe for roasted romaine!
Roasted Romaine Lettuce was introduced to me by my sister-in-law. Her dish is as follows:

I've always loved her, but now I know even more about why my beloved brother got married to her.

The majority of days that fall in autumn, winter, or spring make me crave this recipe because it is so delectable, even on cold and slightly cool days. In addition, I truly enjoy it in the summer when we eat anything grilled.

This dish tastes amazing when eaten exactly as written. Try drizzling with our simple balsamic vinegar reduction and a sprinkle of Parmesan if you're feeling fancy, and see if your taste buds don't explode.

ingredients.

3. Mixed Bean and Lentil Salad Recipe
There are so many different ways to make mixed bean and lentil salad!

with a light, scrumptious dressing, such as this one! You can use pretty much any vegetables and beans you have on hand to combine all the flavors.

If you serve the salad as a side dish with a protein source, you can make it entirely from vegetables. The inclusion of protein-rich legumes in this bean and lentil salad is a great addition if it serves as your main course.

For added convenience, we prefer to use canned beans and lentils, but you can absolutely use precooked beans and lentils.

If you use canned legumes, rinse them well to get rid of any salt that may have been added. Additionally, we advise purchasing low-sodium canned beans. A green leafy salad goes well with a bean and lentil salad. It also tastes great when eaten with crackers or a spoon. Stuffed into a pita or tortilla is a favorite of some people's. We prefer to consume it in lettuce cups. The decision is entirely yours!

This Dressing Chilli powder and cumin are used in the dressing of many bean salads, particularly the American favorite, the three-bean salad. Even though that results in a flavor that is fantastically Southwest, there are times when I just do not want that kind of strong flavor.

Vinegar, garlic, and lime juice make the light and zesty dressing for this bean and lentil salad. Additionally, it is loaded with healthy ingredients. Olive oil and apple cider vinegar are two of these components (in addition to the beans and vegetables, of course).

If you like your bean salads with more or less dressing, you can increase or decrease the amount of dressing.

Is olive oil healthy?
Despite the fact that this myth was prevalent ten years ago, research has virtually dispelled it. The right kind of fat is great for your health!

We adore this article that discusses numerous advantages of olive oil's unsaturated fats. For three years in a row, the Mediterranean Diet has been called the healthiest diet. is due to the emphasis placed on olive oil.

A Mediterranean diet high in olive oil has been shown to significantly lower the risk of heart disease by as much as 30%, according to extensive research.

Is apple cider vinegar beneficial to health?
Many diets could benefit from including vinegar. It adds a lot of flavor to foods without adding a lot of calories or salt. Acetic acid is produced when sugar from apples is fermented. Vinegar is sour because of this acetic acid, which is one of its main active ingredients. Additionally, this probably provides the advantages.

4. Lemon-Garlic Dressing

ItIs healthy to make your own salad dressing? This homemade salad dressing is a must-try if you enjoy salads. In a matter of minutes, it can be mixed up.

Greens and vegetables go well with our lemon-garlic dressing. It won't take much effort to elevate your salads to the next level.

This recipe is so easy to make that you'll never need to buy salad dressing again. It uses ingredients that are healthy and affordable.

Not only are bottled dressings expensive, but they also contain harmful chemicals and preservatives that can easily be avoided by making your own salad dressing. This dressing has a lovely citrus flavor and goes well with a variety of salads.

Olive oil in a homemade salad dressing This homemade salad dressing has a wonderful flavor and coats the salad for the perfect glaze. Olive oil is a good oil for the heart and has many good health benefits.

Many health professionals believe that extra virgin olive oil is the healthiest fat on the planet. The Mediterranean Diet relies heavily on this fat. Olive oil is an effective antioxidant due to its high content of monounsaturated fats and oleic acid, an essential fatty acid for the body.

It also has antioxidants and a lot of Vitamin E, Vitamin K, to help you stay fit and healthy. Olive oil has been shown to protect against a wide range of diseases, including cancer, heart disease, stroke, and Alzheimer's.

How to make this dressing Salad making should be easy and quick!

If you want a dressing that doesn't require much effort, this recipe for homemade salad dressing is the best option. In a bowl, combine a few minced garlic cloves with Dijon mustard, olive oil, lemon, salt, and pepper. That is all.

The dressing gains a lovely aroma from the garlic. The Dijon mustard gives the dish a spicy kick. This is heavenly when combined with olive oil and lemon, and it tastes better than any salad dressing you can buy at the grocery store!

Try out our balsamic vinaigrette if you like this dressing! Please let us know your thoughts!

Ingredients: Juice of one lemon, about 1 tbsp. 3 tbsp. olive oil, 1/2 tsp. Dijon mustard, 1 small, minced garlic clove, salt, and pepper. DIRECTIONS: Whisk together the ingredients in a salad bowl before adding the greens and tossing, or vigorously shake a jar.
can keep for about a week in the refrigerator. The oil will solidify, but you can either remove it at room

temperature for ten to fifteen minutes or run warm water through the jar until it returns to liquid. To recombine, shake.

5. Creamy Slow Cooker Pumpkin Soup Recipe

Savory, Creamy Slow Cooker Pumpkin Soup Is it pumpkin season yet? I must confess that fall is my favorite season. The weather is perfect for wearing sweatshirts in the fall, and the food is the best. Chai tea, applesauce, and pumpkin everything—my personal favorite! Those of you who adore pumpkin, like I do, will appreciate this recipe for creamy pumpkin soup.

With the addition of pumpkin pie spice, this creamy pumpkin soup recipe retains some of the flavors of pumpkin pie but is completely devoid of sweetness, allowing the pumpkin to shine through. A drizzle of maple syrup on top is heaven for those who prefer it sweet. Dressed up just like the picture, I love it spicy. As a main dish, a large bowl of pumpkin soup is perfect with a green salad. It also tastes great in a cup before or after your favorite meal.

For the Kids My children enjoy soup, but not all of them do. Because the consistency of soup is similar to that of pureed baby food, toddlers frequently enjoy it. Offering a wide variety of toppings to children is my favorite way to get them to eat soup. They can thus customize their meal as they please. It's also fun for adults. To make smiley faces frequently, we use topping. Cutting cheese or vegetables into tiny shapes to place on top of the soup adds a fun artistic touch if you feel like it. But you don't have to. Kids will probably be tempted to take a bite when they smell the delicious aroma of this soup cooking. Please comment below. Are you a pumpkin fan? Or do you prefer other flavors of fall? INGREDIENTS: 1 TBSP olive oil, a large diced onion, four cloves of garlic, two 15-ounce cans of pure pumpkin, three cups low-sodium vegetable broth, one 15-ounce can of coconut milk, one TBSP cumin, one teaspoon coriander, one teaspoon pumpkin pie seasoning, and one teaspoon salt (to taste). Seeds, feta cheese, maple syrup (if you prefer it sweet) or cayenne pepper (if you prefer it hot) DIRECTIONS Heat olive oil in a pan over the stove and saute the diced onions until they begin to caramelize a little (5 to 10 minutes). Add the garlic and continue to sauté for a few more minutes, or until it begins to turn a color.

With the exception of the optional toppings, add everything to the Crock Pot. Stir it thoroughly.

Cook for about four hours on low. Enjoy the wonderful aroma in your home!

Puree the soup with an immersion blender until it is very smooth. However, while doing this, be careful not to splash any hot liquid on yourself.) Taste and adjust the seasonings or salt as necessary.

Serve in bowls with any toppings you like.

6. Kale Pomegranate Salad

Healthy dishes Although this salad goes well with heavier meals, it also tastes great on its own. It is loaded with winter foods that are simple to obtain from your neighbourhood grocery store. Winter is when kale, pomegranates, and pears are in season, so they are typically more affordable and have more health benefits. Did you know that December is designated as National Pear Month by the USDA? Another reason to savour this delectable dish! One of the healthiest vegetables you can consume is kale. Antioxidants in kale are to blame for everything from slowing down ageing to lowering your risk of cancer. Tell Popeye that a cup of raw kale, like the kale in this salad, has 2 grams of protein. It also contains 200% of your daily value of vitamin A, calcium, iron, fibre, and over 600% of your daily value of vitamin K. It is regrettable that the average American consumes very little kale. Check out how delicious this fantastic winter salad can be!

Ingredients: 10 ounces of fresh kale; 1/2 small pomegranate (approximately 3/4 cup of seeds); 1 chopped pear; 3 ounces of crumbled goat cheese; 1/2 cup chopped pecans (or walnuts).
4 tablespoons olive oil 1 to 2 tablespoons pure maple syrup (start with 1 and work your way up) 1 teaspoon dijon mustard 2 tablespoons apple cider vinegar 1/4 teaspoon salt (optional) DIRECTIONS Thinly slice the kale and remove the tough ribs and stems. Put everything in a big bowl.
Dress the salad: Today, combine everything in a bowl or blender—oil, maple syrup, mustard, and vinegar.
Reserving approximately one-fourth of the dressing for guests to add at the table, drizzle the majority of the dressing over the kale in the bowl. Massage the

coated kale with your hands for a few minutes to begin to soften the leaves.

Remove the pomegranate's seeds (see our guide for instructions!) Pears should be chopped.

Add the goat cheese, chopped pears, pomegranate seeds, and pecans to the large bowl with the kale. Reserve some of each for each diner's salad bowl. To coat, gently toss. Adjust the salt to taste.

Add the dressed salad to the bowls of each diner. Cheese, the remaining seeds, and pecans complete the top. With the extra dressing, serve.

7.Watercress, Tomato, and Butternut Squash Soup

INGREDIENTS 2 TBSP olive oil 2 large tomatoes, seeded and chopped, 1 small onion, 1 clove garlic, 2 carrots, chopped, 1 butternut squash, peeled and chopped, 1 medium potato, peeled and chopped, 1 bunch watercress, including stems, 2 cups reduced-sodium vegetable broth, 4 cups water, 1/3 cup frozen corn kernels, defrosted

Stirring frequently, cook the tomatoes, onion, and garlic for 12 minutes.

Squash, potatoes, watercress, and broth are all options.

Ingredients should be brought to a boil, then simmer covered for 30 minutes.

Return to a boil with the water, reduce the heat, and simmer covered for ten minutes.

After removing the saucepan from the heat, allow the soup to cool to room temperature. Puree, either by putting portions of the soup into a blender or using an immersion blender.

Add salt and pepper to taste to the soup. If necessary, reheat. Use the corn kernels as a garnish. Yum!

8. Beet Goat Cheese Salad

This Beet Goat Cheese Salad Recipe is a great option for a light lunch or dinner. This Beet Goat Cheese Salad is your answer! This salad is a real hit thanks to the zingy homemade dressing, the healthy fats from the cheese and walnuts, and the fiber from the lettuce and beets.

This salad is incredibly simple to prepare. Simply arrange the ingredients and salad in bowls. In a small bowl, combine the citrus dressing. Apply the dressing to the salad. Amazing! For two ways to cook fresh beets, see the notes below. Or, you can do as we frequently do and buy a container of beets that have already been cooked. Wash any canned goods thoroughly.

This recipe serves two to three people. How much salad you want to eat is everything! You could also make small portions and eat them as a side salad or as a salad before dinner.

How to Cook Fresh Beets There are a few different approaches you can take if you have never cooked fresh beets before.

Bake them. Cut fresh beets in half and arrange them on a baking sheet lined with aluminum foil while the oven is preheating to 400 degrees F. Roast for about an hour, or until the beet's middle can be easily cut through. After allowing to cool completely, peel and slice the fruit. Beets can turn anything they touch pink and are very messy! Use gloves or forks when slicing to avoid pinking your hands!

Boil them. Over medium heat, bring a big pot of water to a boil. Put the beets in and cook them for about 40 minutes in boiling water. Remove the water. Let the beets cool down. Then slice and peel. Again, beets can turn anything they touch pink and are very messy! Use gloves or forks when slicing to avoid pinking your hands!

Pre-cooked beets in a can, bag, or jar are another option. Check to see that there is no sugar added. Additionally, we always advise washing any canned foods to remove excess salt. This is the path we frequently take!

Ingredients: 3 cups romaine or arugula greens, 4 large beets (or 1 can of pre-cooked beets), 5 clementine oranges, 1/2 cup walnuts, and 1/2 cup goat or feta cheese.

Directions (To use fresh beets, either roast them for one hour at 400 degrees or boil them for about 40 minutes in a large pot of boiling water.) 1/4 cup olive oil 2 TBSP orange juice 1/4 TBSP Dijon mustard Salt and pepper to taste (we recommend 1/8 tsp of each). Slice them after they have cooled for both methods. For more, see the notes.)

Clementines should be separated. Grate the feta or goat cheese.

Whisk together the olive oil, orange juice, mustard, honey, salt, and pepper to make the salad dressing.

In bowls, add the salad greens. Cheese, beets, oranges, and walnuts should be topped. Apply dressing to the dish. Enjoy right away!

9. Kale Salad with Quinoa

A Delicious and Complete Meal:

Whole grains, protein, and healthy fats are all well-balanced in this tasty Kale Salad with Quinoa. It also contains phytochemicals, antioxidants, a variety of essential vitamins, minerals, and nutrients. If you're like us, one of your goals is to include more green foods in your diet. A mouthwatering way to do it is with this salad! This is a delicious lunch, light dinner, or smaller side dish that is packed with whole grains, vitamins from the fruits and vegetables, and healthy fats. Try bringing this to a potluck and everyone will rave about how delicious and healthy it is! Gluten-free, dairy-free, and vegan are all ingredients in this salad. Make sure your quinoa has been labeled accordingly.

Other advantages for health include:

Avocado is a good source of potassium and monounsaturated fat.

Quinoa is a whole grain that contains all seven essential amino acids and is a complete vegan protein.

Kale is loaded with nutrients that fight cancer: antioxidants and the vitamins K, C, and A.

Antioxidants, which are nutrients that are known to lower the risk of cancer, are abundant in pomegranates.

Antioxidants and alpha linolenic acid (ALA), the plant-based form of omega 3, are abundant in walnuts.

Making this Quick Kale Salad with Quinoa This salad is also incredibly simple to prepare. Since seeding the pomegranate will take the most time, we recommend purchasing it pre-seeded if you are short on time. Check out our guide on how to seed them correctly if you want to give it a shot. The second part of this salad that takes any time to prepare is the quinoa. This salad is often made with leftover grains. Because it is a complete protein, we chose quinoa for this dish. Brown rice, which is shown in the picture, is another delicious option. The dressing can be mixed quickly with a whisk. It will keep for a few days in your refrigerator if you don't use all of the dressing! If the dressing separates, simply stir it back together after letting it sit for a few minutes. It tastes so good on many different salads. Don't miss this for more delicious soups and salads!

Ingredients: One and a half cups cooked quinoa (leftovers are great!).

1 cup chopped kale, 1 pomegranate that has been seeded, 1/2 cup chopped walnuts, 1 avocado, 1 pound cooked chicken that has been diced, 1/4 cup lime juice, 2 TBSP orange juice, 1 TBSP honey, 1/3 cup cilantro, and the directions. Make sure that everything is chopped and diced.

Mix the ingredients for the dressing together: honey, orange juice, lime juice, and cilantro.

In a bowl, combine all of the ingredients for the salad.

Add the dressing to the ingredients for the salad.

Enjoy!

10. Tahini Chicken Salad

The Mediterranean Diet allows dairy in moderation, particularly dairy products with additional health benefits like kefir and yoghurt. However, lactose intolerance or personal preference may lead some individuals to avoid dairy products. Dairy can be found in some recipes for chicken salad. Dairy will be present throughout the recipe if the dressing is made with yoghurt or cream, or if the mix-ins contain any kind of cheese like feta. However, this recipe for tahini chicken salad does not contain milk, lactose, or dairy. You won't have to worry about it because you don't eat dairy.

How to Make Vegetarian or Vegan Chicken Salad Is it possible to make this salad vegan by omitting the chicken? Yes, definitely! This chicken salad may be even better than a mayonnaise-based alternative for non-meat eaters due to the protein-rich Tahini. The proportion of dressing to salad will be off after you remove the chicken. Reduce the amount of dressing by half or add more to the salad. You can increase the size of the salad by adding more celery, apples, or new additions like grape halves, chopped carrots, or chopped yellow bell peppers.

Ingredients: 2 and a half cups cooked chicken, 1 and a half cups chopped celery (about 4 to 5 ribs), 1 cup chopped apples, 1/2 cup dried cranberries, 2 teaspoons dried dill, 1/4 cup tahini, 1/4 teaspoon garlic powder, 1/8 teaspoon onion powder, 1 TBSP apple cider vinegar, 3 TBSP hot water, salt and pepper to taste (we recommend 1/8 tsp of each), honey* (if your tahini is too bitter, adding a bit of honey will make it taste better) DIRECTIONS Make sure your chicken is cooked and chopped. If not, proceed with cooking and chopping.

Chop all of the mix-ins into bite-sized pieces that are roughly the same size. In a large bowl, combine everything, including the chicken and dill.

Make the dressing now. Mix the tahini, garlic, onion, and any additional salt and pepper in a separate bowl. Whisk in the 1 TBSP apple cider for a few minutes to incorporate it thoroughly. To make a dressing, continue to whisk in hot water. Let's taste. If your tahini is bitter, add some honey to sweeten it up and thoroughly stir.

In a large bowl, pour the dressing over the salad and thoroughly stir to combine. Enjoy

11.Cozy Vegetable Soup

This recipe for vegetable soup almost guarantees success. Whatever vegetables you have, the base soup, which is made of broth, diced tomatoes, tomato sauce, and seasoning, will be delicious. You don't have to stick to what's written here. Is cabbage on the verge of spoiling? Toss it in with the celery and chop it up. Have leftover lentils, carrots, or broccoli? In the soup, they will all be delicious! Since the vegetables soften naturally, even frozen vegetables work perfectly.

The frozen vegetables should be thawed before being added to the soup to prevent the soup from becoming too watery. You can also play around with the amount of liquid, depending on how you like it. This soup will be more "soup-like" if it contains more liquid, while if it contains less, it will have more of the consistency of chili. You can make it exactly as written or experiment with different flavors and spices. Make a pot for yourself, and you'll be glad you did. Now, tell us in the comments section if you eat soup for breakfast!

Ingredients: 2 tablespoons of olive oil, a large onion, a large red bell pepper, celery, up to 2 cups of celery, a 28-ounce can of diced tomatoes, 4 ounces of tomato sauce, 6 cups of low-sodium chicken or vegetable broth (you could also use 4 cups of broth and 2 cups of water), 1 tablespoon of Italian seasoning, up to 1 teaspoon of red pepper flakes (optional), for spiciness, 2 cans of beans, any variety You do not need to chop the spinach because it will wilt; all you need to do is make sure there are no large leaves.)

In a large pot, heat the oil, garlic, and onions over medium heat. 3 to 5 minutes or until the onions start to brown.

Cook another 5 minutes, adding the celery and peppers, until everything starts to soften.

Add chicken broth, Italian seasoning, tomatoes (including their liquid), tomato sauce, and, if desired, red pepper flakes to the pot. Everything should simmer for about fifteen minutes.

Add spinach and cans of beans that have been well drained. Allow the spinach to wilt and everything to heat up while the pot continues to cook.

Taste, adjust the salt and pepper, and remove from the heat. Keep warm. Keeps well in the refrigerator for several days!

12. Turkey Chilli Recipe

SPICES FOR CHILLI RECIPES

Chili can also be made in any way you want. You can adapt the spices to suit your family by substituting different vegetables, beans, meat, or other vegetarian protein. We keep our main chilli pot pretty tame because we have a couple of young children in the house. From a spice standpoint, this turkey chili recipe is pretty mild). I season mine with hot sauce and sometimes cayenne pepper after it has been cooked. I adore the heat! Try increasing the amount of chilli powder to 4 TBSP and adding a few pinches of cayenne if your family enjoys a lot of heat. I would suggest sticking with the straightforward original chilli recipe if your family doesn't like spice.

ADDITIONAL INGREDIENTS FOR THE TURKEY CHILI There are numerous additional ingredients that could make the turkey chili even more delectable. I love to stir some fresh greens into the chilli until they wilt at the very end, especially spinach, but any kind will do. Chopped cauliflower is an additional excellent addition. To ensure that it blends in well with the other pieces, I like to chop it very small. Chilli with pumpkin is another family favorite! However, that's a recipe for another time. Do whatever comes to mind. Utilize everything in your refrigerator.

TURKEY CHILLI IN THE CROCK POT We adore the crock pot around here, as you may know. I love knowing that dinner will be ready when dinnertime arrives by dumping all of my ingredients into the pot at the beginning of the day. The perfect example of a quick, healthy, and delicious meal is this turkey chilli in the crock pot. However, you can also prepare this chilli over the stove! The process is basically the same. Follow the instructions to cook the turkey and onion. After that, sauté the zucchini and peppers for a few minutes. Include the tomatoes, broth, and all of the spices. Everything should simmer for ten to fifteen minutes. To prevent the beans and corn from becoming mushy, I prefer to add them last. Tada! For this delicious dinner, either method will work perfectly. Simply keep in mind all of the toppings. Like soup? Try Pumpkin Soup and Vegetable Soup, two of our other favorites. Please let us know how you like this slow cooker chilli recipe

! INGREDIENTS 2 teaspoons olive oil 1 chopped onion 4 minced garlic cloves 1 chopped zucchini (and peeled if desired) 1 chopped bell pepper (any color) 1 pound lean ground turkey 3 TBSP chilli powder 2 tsp cumin 1 tsp dried oregano 1/2 tsp salt (to taste) 2 canned fire-roasted diced tomatoes, with the liquid 1/2 cups chicken or vegetable broth (reduced-sodium preferred) 1 can beans, Optional toppings: 1 cup cooked quinoa SOUR CREAM, cilantro, avocado, and other

ingredients DIRECTIONS

Chop all of your vegetables roughly to size.

In a skillet, combine the chopped onions and garlic with the olive oil. Stir frequently while cooking over medium-high heat to avoid burning. Increase the heat to medium when the onions have begun to caramelize.

Sauté the ground turkey for about 7 minutes until browned.

Add everything to the slow cooker, stirring a few times to combine the chili.

Cook for 3 to 4 hours on high or 6-7 hours on low.

Stir the quinoa into the crockpot at the end if using it.

Warm up in bowls and top with a lot of toppings!

Chapter four
29 Fish and sea food

1. Deep-fried, oven-baked fish with herb-infused
Breadcrumbs are the ultimate equaliser. It transforms any raw ingredient, no matter how nutritious it may be, into nutritional waste. In addition, have you ever noticed that all fried foods have the same flavour? Don't you think so? Try to distinguish between the various types of fried seafood when you order the 1,650-calorie Admiral's Feast from Red Lobster.) Fish has a flavour that is exciting and complex, and it is full of nutrients that are healthy and energising. Therefore, why doom them in a greasy deep fryer? Our healthy fish topped with herbed breadcrumbs steps in to save the day here. This oven-baked fish still has butter in it, but it has a breadcrumb topping that gives it the crunch and richness of deep fried food without affecting the fish's flavor or nutrition. It also has more than half the calories.

4 halibut fillets or other flaky white fish, such as cod or swordfish, (4–6 oz each) (Thinner fillets like

catfish and tilapia are likely to overcook before the breadcrumbs are toasted, but any thick white fish fillet will be perfect). You'll need 2 slices of white bread or 1 English muffin, split. 2 tablespoons chopped fresh parsley. 1 teaspoon fresh thyme leaves.

To taste, salt and black pepper 2 tablespoons softened butter. HOW TO MAKE IT Preheat the oven to 450 degrees Fahrenheit.

In a food processor, pulse the bread, parsley, and thyme until you have small but not superfine breadcrumbs. Here, you need a little texture.

Salt and pepper the fish on all sides before placing it on a baking sheet.

Press the herbed breadcrumbs into the butter to ensure that they adhere to the fish after coating the tops with a thin layer of softened butter.

Bake for about 20 minutes, or until the fish flakes when gently pressed with a fingertip.

Eat This Tip: If you need breadcrumbs but don't want to use gluten, look for a box of panko breadcrumbs at your local grocery store (Ian's is a well-known brand). Even without the gluten, you'll still enjoy the crunch.

2. Low-Calorie Baked Fish and Chips Recipe

We adore everything about the concept of fish and chips—the pile of crispy potatoes, the tartar sauce or malt vinegar on the side, and the crunch of the batter that plays off the tender bite of the fish. This recipe is a lighthearted ode to the English staple, which is a well-known dish on a menu. We coat cod fillets with crushed salt and vinegar potato chips before baking them until they are crispy and golden brown, bringing the whole fish and chips experience together in one bite. The most regrettable aspect of fish and chips is the only thing it leaves out. all of the extra fat from the deep fryer. However, you are not required to forego the chips entirely! If you want to serve real chips on the side, we recommend smoked paprika potato chips or crispy, oven-baked fries. This way, you can skip the deep fryer and reduce your waistline at the same time!

4 cod fillets, each 6 ounces, are required. 1 cup nonfat buttermilk, Tabasco to taste, 3/4 cup panko bread crumbs, 1/4 cup crushed salt and vinegar chips, salt and black pepper to taste, 2 tablespoons olive oil mayonnaise, 2 tablespoons Greek yogurt, 1 lemon juice, 2 tablespoons chopped pickles, 1

tablespoon capers, and 1 teaspoon Dijon mustard. Refrigerate for 20 minutes to marinate.

The oven should be heated to 400°F.

Season with a few pinches of salt and black pepper in a shallow baking dish the crushed chips and bread crumbs.

Remove the fish from the buttermilk one piece at a time and roll it in the coating before patting the mixture onto the fish with your fingers.

Place the coated fish on a baking sheet-mounted rack. Bake for about 15 minutes, or until the fish flakes easily with your finger's gentle pressure and the coating is nicely browned and crunchy.

In a mixing bowl, combine the Dijon, mayonnaise, yogurt, lemon juice, pickles, and capers while the fish bakes.

On the side, spoon some tartar sauce over the fish.

3. Blackened Fish Sandwich with Avocado and Cabbage Recipe

The standard fish sandwich in the United States is a slab of heavily processed mystery seafood that has been breaded, deep fried, and stuffed into a huge, squishy roll. The seafood is then covered in a tartar-like sauce. For something that is supposed to be healthy, you lose between 600 and 800 calories and the majority of your daily sodium intake. Fresh tilapia fillets, blackened frying, tartar sauce made with creamy avocado and crunchy cabbage make up our fish sandwich. This blackened fish sandwich has a lot of flavor, so you won't miss the mystery meat substitute you're used to.

1 cup plain Greek-style yogurt 1 teaspoon sriracha 1 lime juice 1 tablespoon canola oil 4 whole-wheat sesame seed buns 4 tilapia or catfish fillets (6 ounces each) 1 teaspoon blackening seasoning 1 avocado, pitted, peeled, and sliced 2 cups shredded red cabbage Pickled onions Place aside.

In a large cast-iron skillet, heat the oil to a high temperature. The fish fillets should be rubbed both sides with a lot of the seasoning for blackening.

Add the fish to the pan when the oil is smoking, and cook for three minutes, uncovered, until a dark crust forms.

Cook the fillets on the other side for an additional 2 to 3 minutes, or until the fish flakes easily with your finger pressure.

Toast the buns, cut side up, under the broiler while the fish is cooking. Split the cabbage and avocado among the buns. Onions, yogurt sauce, and hot fish should be served on top.

4. Recipe for Seared Ahi Tuna with a Ginger-Scallion Sauce

We love ahi tuna for its abundance of lean protein and heart- and brain-healthy omega-3 fatty acids, but what we love most about this fish is that even a novice cook can prepare it perfectly in less than five minutes. That is correct; you have this. A high-heat pan, a little oil, some salt and pepper, and that's all there is to it. To make this a more substantial and nutritious dish, we add bok choy, but any green vegetable (spinach, broccoli, asparagus, kale, string beans, etc.) will do. will work. However, we can assure you that the ubiquitous ginger-scallion sauce, which is good enough to transform an old pair of socks into a delectably memorable meal, should not be skipped.

1 bunch scallions, with the bottoms removed, finely chopped; 2 tablespoons fresh ginger, peeled and grated; 1 tablespoon low-sodium soy sauce; 3 tablespoons peanut oil; 1 tablespoon rice wine vinegar; 16 ounces ahi or other high-quality tuna steaks; salt and pepper to taste; 12 pound shiitake

mushrooms, with the stems removed; 1 pound baby bok choy, with the stems removed.

HOW TO MAKE IT

Place aside. This can be made ahead of time and stored in the refrigerator because even 30 minutes of sitting time allows the flavors to marry well.)

In a large sauté pan or cast-iron skillet, heat the remaining oil.

The tuna should be generously seasoned with black pepper and salt.

Add the tuna to the pan when the oil is lightly smoking and sear for 2 minutes on each side until it is deeply browned. Remove.

Add the shiitake mushrooms to the same hot pan while the tuna rests (add more oil if the pan is dry).

Add the bok choy after cooking for 2 to 3 minutes until it is lightly browned. Bok choy should be lightly wilted after another two to three minutes of cooking. Sprinkle with salt and pepper to taste.

The tuna should be cut into thick strips. Divide the mushrooms and bok choy among four hot plates.

The ginger-scallion sauce should be drizzled over the tuna slices.

5. Tuna and Avocado Fish Taco Recipe Ground beef, crunchy shells, and shredded cheese are the staples of the typical American taco night. That's fine, but other types of fish and meat can provide more flavor for a fraction of the calories. Example A: tuna ahi. The flavors are hard to beat, especially when topped with a spicy slaw and a few pickled onions, and the combination of silky-rare tuna and creamy avocado packs a lot of healthy fat into the palm of your hand. Avoid the fried variety: Your new fish taco recipe is here.

4 cups shredded cabbage, 2 tablespoons olive oil-based mayonnaise, 1 lime wedge for serving, 2 tablespoons canned chipotle pepper, salt and black pepper to taste, 2 tablespoons canola or olive oil, 12 ounces fresh ahi or other high-quality tuna, 8 corn tortillas, 1 ripe avocado, pitted, peeled, and sliced Pickled red onions, hot sauce.

HOW TO MAKE IT
Add salt and pepper to taste. Put the slaw away. To allow the flavors to combine, do this at least 15 minutes before cooking.)

In a large sauté pan made of stainless steel or cast iron, heat the oil to medium-high heat.

Use a lot of black pepper and salt to season the tuna.

Add the tuna to the hot oil and sear for 2 minutes on each side, until the tuna has developed a nice crust but the inside is still rare.

Heat the tortillas until they are lightly crisp on the outside while the pan is still hot.

Planks of thin tuna should be sliced.

Top each tortilla with avocado slices, slaw, and pickled onions. Divide among the tortillas.

Hot sauce and lime wedges are optional.

6. Asian-Inspired Tuna Burger with Wasabi Mayo

Tuna is a firm, meaty fish that is ideal for burgers. We love making tuna burgers for a meal that is packed with protein. A quick pulse in the food processor or even a small amount of fine chopping is all that is required. In either case, the fish should be extremely cold to prevent the proteins from clumping together. The ground tuna that results can be shaped into patties and dressed in a plethora of ways. (Salmon works just as well if you don't want to eat tuna.)

Additionally, if you top your burger with a spicy wasabi mayo, you'll get a burger that packs a punch in every bite. This is very different from your typical burger!

1 lb fresh tuna, 4 minced scallions, 1 teaspoon minced fresh ginger, 1 tablespoon low-sodium soy sauce, 1 teaspoon toasted sesame oil, canola oil for grilling, 2 tablespoons olive oil mayonnaise, 12 teaspoons prepared wasabi (from powder or in premade paste), 4 whole-wheat sesame buns, split and lightly toasted, 1 cup sliced cucumber, lightly salted, 2 cups mixed baby greens.

HOW TO MAKE IT

Pulse the tuna in a food processor to the consistency of ground beef, working in batches if necessary. Be careful not to go overboard; Pulsing it just enough to make patties is all you need to do.)

Add the scallions, ginger, soy sauce, and sesame oil to a mixing bowl. Make four patties of equal size.

Before grilling, place in the fridge for at least 10 minutes to firm up.

Pre-heat a grill pan or well-oiled grill.

Add the patties to the hot pan and cook for 2 to 3 minutes on each side until they are browned on the outside and still medium rare in the middle.

These burgers are more delicate than beef burgers, so flip and handle them carefully.

Spread the wasabi-mayonnaise mixture evenly over the tops of the buns.

The burgers should be placed on top of the cucumber and greens, and the tops of the buns should be used as a crown.

7.Recipe for Quick and Easeful Italian Tuna Melt
the tuna melt: Has any sandwich ever wasted more opportunities than this dodgy mess? Aren't the memories visceral and odourless? They don't have to be, anyway. Let's re-create this tasty, quick meal!

The majority of establishments' recipe reveals everything: Typically, they use 1 part tuna to 2 parts mayo. The majority of the mayo in our version is replaced by a significantly healthier supporting cast that enhances flavor without adding additional fat: olives, onions, pesto, and juice from one lemon This means that when you eat it, you can taste something other than fat and feel something other than fat.

You'll need 2 cans of tuna, each 5 ounces, drained; 1 small red onion, diced; 1/4 cup chopped green olives; 2 tablespoons olive oil mayonnaise; 2 tablespoons bottled pesto; 1 tablespoon rinsed and chopped capers; 1 lemon juice; 8 slices whole-wheat bread; 2 ounces fresh mozzarella, sliced; you can also use low-fat shredded mozzarella; 1 large tomato, sliced; and about 1 teaspoon olive oil.

HOW TO MAKE IT
Heat a nonstick or cast-iron pan on medium heat.
Apply a light coating of olive oil to each sandwich and cook for 2 to 3 minutes on each side, or until the cheese is melted and the bread is toasty.

8. Crispy Chipotle Shrimp Quesadilla
Careful crisping of the tortilla's exterior is the key to a world-class quesadilla. In years of analyzing nutritional information, we have never discovered a restaurant quesadilla with fewer than 900 calories and 50 grams of fat because restaurants compensate

for their sloppy cooking by adding more cheese and oil. There is a lot of cheese in this quesadilla, but thanks to the abundance of spicy shrimp and caramelized vegetables and the shattering crust of the tortilla, we can cut fat in this recipe without sacrificing flavor.

4 large whole-wheat tortillas 2 cups shredded Monterey Jack cheese Salsa Guacamole WHAT YOU NEED: 8 oz. medium shrimp that have been peeled and deveined; 12 tbsp. canola oil; 1 medium onion that has been sliced; 1 red or yellow bell pepper that has been sliced; salt and black pepper to taste. HOW TO MAKE IT: Combine the shrimp with the orange juice, chipotle pepper, and garlic. Give it a 15-minute marinade.

In a large sauté pan or cast-iron skillet, heat the oil to a medium-high temperature.

Add the onion and pepper and cook for about 10 minutes, or until lightly charred on the outside, until the oil is lightly smoking.

Place the shrimp in the middle of the pan and push the vegetables to the edges of the pan.

Sauté for about ten minutes or until cooked through.

To taste, season with salt and pepper. Turn off the heat.

Heat a separate nonstick pan over medium-low heat and coat it with cooking spray, oil, or butter. Layer one tortilla on top of the other, top with half of the shrimp mixture and a second tortilla, and sprinkle with half of the cheese.

Flip and cook for an additional 2 to 3 minutes, or until the bottom is extremely crisp.

Serve the quesadillas with salsa and, if desired, a little guacamole. Cut the quesadillas into wedges.

9. Southern-Style Shrimp and Grits Recipe

1 tbsp canola oil 1 cup diced cooked turkey kielbasa 4 scallions, whites, and greens separated, chopped 1 clove garlic, minced 8 oz fresh mushrooms (button, cremini, or shiitake), stems removed, sliced 1 pound shrimp, peeled and deveined 12 tsp cayenne pepper 12 oz quick-cooking grits 1 Include the Kielbasa cook until just lightly browned for a few minutes. Include the mushrooms, garlic, and whites of scallions.

3 to 4 minutes or until the mushrooms are lightly browned.

Continue cooking the shrimp until they are just pink and firm to the touch after adding them. Add the broth and cook for an additional 3 minutes, stirring frequently, until the shrimp are cooked through and the liquid has been reduced by half. Add cayenne, salt, and pepper to taste.

Cook the grits as directed on the package while the shrimp are cooking. Add the cheese and season with salt and pepper when they are thick and creamy.

Using the scallion greens as a garnish, divide the shrimp and grits among four bowls.

10. A Shrimp Lo Mein Recipe

That's Better Than Takeout! You'll need 12 ounces of lo mein noodles, 1 tablespoon of peanut or vegetable oil, 2 minced cloves of garlic, 1 tablespoon of grated fresh ginger, 4 scallions, whites and greens separated, chopped, 4 ounces of shiitake mushrooms, 2 medium carrots, cut into thin slices, 12 red bell pepper, sliced, and 4 lb medium shrimp, peeled and deveined.

Heat the oil to a high temperature in a wok or large skillet.

Stir-fry the garlic, ginger, and scallion whites for 30 seconds, until lightly golden, when the oil is lightly smoking.

Using a metal spatula, cook the mushrooms, carrots, and bell pepper for 3 to 4 minutes more, making sure they move almost continuously.

Cook the shrimp, tossing them in, until they are just pink and slightly firm.

In the pan, add the cooked noodles, oyster sauce, and soy sauce.

Continue to cook for one to two more minutes, or until the sauce has thickened and covers the noodles lightly.

Place the scallion greens on top of the mixture and divide it among the four plates.

Eat This Tip to Cut Calories: Forget the Fork Our brains influence our appetites nearly as much as our stomachs do, and it's easier than you think to fool both. The use of chopsticks rather than a fork is one option. Chopsticks are culturally acceptable because they force you to work for your food, allowing your brain to send signals to your stomach that it is full before you overeat. The remainder can then be used for leftovers. Take into consideration the in-house takeout leftovers!

11.Low-Calorie Shrimp Fra Diavolo Recipe

12 Tbsp olive oil, 2 tsp red pepper flakes, 1 small chopped onion, 2 minced cloves of garlic, 1/4 tsp

dried oregano or thyme, 1 can (28 oz.) crushed tomatoes, 1 cup dry white wine, 8 oz. spaghetti, 2 tbsp chopped flat-leaf parsley HOW TO MAKE IT Season the shrimp with salt and pepper. In a large sauté pan or skillet, heat the oil to a medium temperature.

Cook the shrimp for one to two minutes, or until just firm, adding them. Place on a plate.

In the pan, add the oregano, onion, garlic, and pepper flakes; cook the onions until they are soft.

Simmer for ten to fifteen minutes before adding the wine and tomatoes.

Cook the spaghetti as directed on the package in the meantime.

Return the drain to the pot.

Salt and pepper are used to season the sauce.

Mix the sauce with the cooked shrimp. Toss the pasta in the pan.

With the parsley on top, serve.

Eat This Tip We enjoy canned tomatoes for their flavor just as much as we do for their affordability and nutritional content (they contain more lycopene than fresh tomatoes). Additionally, Muir Glen's organic fire-roasted canned tomatoes are our favorite. They have a beautiful smoky flavor and a faint char when they come out of the can, making your sauce taste like it's been simmering for days.

12.Oven-Roasted Shrimp Cocktail Recipe

1 lb. raw shrimp that have been peeled and deveined; 1 tbsp. olive oil; 1 tsp. Old Bay seasoning (optional); salt and black pepper to taste; 1 tbsp. prepared horseradish; 1 tsp. sriracha or another hot sauce; 1 tbsp. ketchup; 1 tbsp.

Toss the shrimp with the salt and pepper, olive oil, and Old Bay, if using, on a baking sheet. The shrimp should be pink and just firm when baked for about 5 minutes.

Combine the horseradish, sriracha, ketchup, and lemon juice while the shrimp is cooking.

Taste the spice and adjust it to your liking. With the shrimp, serve.

Eat This Tip: How to devein shrimp The vein that runs down the back of the shrimp is actually the digestive tract, so removing it before cooking is a good idea. Fortunately, it's also very easy.

13.Versatile Shrimp and Mango Summer Roll Recipe

YOU WILL NEED: 1 tbsp chunky peanut butter, 1 tbsp sugar, 2 tbsp fish sauce, 2 tbsp rice wine vinegar, plus more for the noodles. 2 oz vermicelli or thin rice noodles (capellini or angel hair pasta also works) 8 sheets of rice paper. 12 lb cooked medium shrimp, each sliced in half. 12 red bell pepper, thinly sliced. 1 Combine thoroughly by stirring. Set aside the peanut sauce.

Follow the directions on the package to cook the noodles.

To prevent sticking, drain and toss with a few shakes of vinegar.

Dip a piece of rice paper in warm water for a few seconds until it becomes just soft and pliable.

On a cutting board, place the paper. Top with noodles, three or four shrimp halves, bell pepper, mango, scallion, and a few whole cilantro leaves, leaving a 12" space at each end of the wrapper.

Roll the rice paper tightly like a burrito after folding the ends toward the center. Continue with the remaining seven wrappers. With the peanut sauce, serve.

14. A Spanish Garlic Shrimp Recipe You'll Need: 14 cup olive oil, 6 thinly sliced cloves of garlic, 14 teaspoon red pepper flakes, 1 lb medium shrimp that have been peeled and deveined, 12 teaspoon smoked paprika, salt and pepper to taste, and 14 cup chopped fresh parsley.

Cook slowly for about 5 minutes, being careful not to burn, until very soft and caramelized.

Add the salt and smoked paprika-seasoned shrimp to the pan.

Cook, turning once, just until cooked through, about 4 minutes total.

Serve with bread to dip in the garlic oil and sprinkle with parsley.

15. A Healthy Shrimp and Spinach Salad with Warm Bacon

You'll Need: 8 ounces shrimp, peeled and deveined (shrimp is one of nature's greatest sources of selenium, a micromineral that helps reduce joint inflammation and fight off free radicals that cause cancer).

Salt and black pepper to taste 2 tablespoons pine nuts, 1 tablespoon Dijon mustard, 3 tablespoons red wine vinegar Olive oil (optional) 1 bag of baby spinach, 6 ounces, 2 sliced hard-boiled eggs In 5 to 7 minutes, cook the bacon until crispy. Transfer to a plate and reserve on a paper towel using a slotted spoon.

Cook the mushrooms and onion in the hot pan for three minutes or until they begin to brown. Add the pine nuts and the salt-and-pepper-seasoned shrimp to the hot pan.

Shrimp cook faster than nearly any other protein, and nobody likes shrimp that are overcooked. Cook the shrimp for no more than four minutes.

In the pan, combine the vinegar and mustard; Add salt and pepper to taste. Olive oil can be added to the pan if it appears to be dry.

Top the eggs and spinach on four plates with some of the pan's liquid and the hot shrimp mixture. Sprinkle the bacon on top.

16.Baked Crab Cakes with Mango-Avocado Salsa

You'll need a 16-ounce can of jumbo lump crab meat, 2 tablespoons minced jalapeo, 2 chopped scallions, 12 cups minced red bell pepper, 1 lightly beaten egg, 2 teaspoons Dijon mustard, 1 lemon, 14 teaspoons Old Bay seasoning, 12 teaspoons salt, and 34 cups bread crumbs. Mango-avocado salsa (You can make your Who doesn't like mangoes? Instead, make your own healthy tartar by combining chopped pickles, capers, and fresh lemon juice with equal parts plain yogurt.)

Preheat the oven to 425°F. HOW TO MAKE IT
Mix everything gently, except for the 12 cups of bread crumbs. Form eight patties from the crab mixture using your hands.
Roll each crab cake in the remaining bread crumbs on a plate to coat them evenly and lightly.
Place the cakes on a baking sheet or baking dish coated with non-stick cooking spray as they form.
Use the palm of your hand to press the patties down into an even disk the size of a small hockey puck if they are misshaped.
12 to 15 minutes or until golden brown on the outside Scoop some mango-avocado salsa on top.

17.Spicy Grilled Calamari Salad
You'll Need: 1 pound cleaned squid, tentacles saved for another use, 12 tablespoons peanut or canola oil, salt, and black pepper to taste, 1 lime juice, 1 tablespoon fish sauce, 1 tablespoon sugar, and 2 tablespoons chili garlic sauce (preferably sambal

oelek). It is simple to substitute baby arugula or even a few handfuls of basil leaves here.)

1 matchstick-sized cucumber, peeled and seeded; 1 medium tomato, chopped; 12 very thinly sliced red onions; and 1 cup roasted peanuts. HOW TO MAKE IT

Season the squid bodies generously with salt and a lot of black pepper after tossing them with the oil.

Add the squid to the grill when it is very hot and cook for about 5 minutes until it is lightly charred all over.

In a mixing bowl, whisk together the chilli sauce, sugar, lime juice, and fish sauce.

The grilled squid should be cut into 12" rings.

Toss the squid, watercress, cucumber, tomato, onion, peanuts, and dressing in a salad bowl.

Split the salad between four plates.

18.Easy Scallops with Chimichurri Recipe

1 lb. large sea scallops, 12 teaspoons salt, 2 tablespoons red wine vinegar, 1 cup chopped fresh parsley, 2 cloves minced garlic, and 3 tablespoons olive oil. Black pepper to taste. HOW TO MAKE IT: Microwave the water and salt in a bowl for 30

seconds. After thoroughly mixing in the vinegar, parsley, garlic, and pepper flakes, stir in the salt.

Whisk as you slowly drizzle in two tablespoons of olive oil. The chimichurri can be used right away, but it's best to let the flavors marry for at least 20 minutes; It will keep for three days in the refrigerator covered.

In a large skillet, heat the remaining 1 tablespoon of oil to medium-high. Salt and pepper the scallops on both sides after thoroughly drying them with paper towels.

Add the scallops to the hot oil and cook for 2 to 3 minutes on each side, stirring occasionally, until a deep brown crust forms. Cook on the flip side for one to two more minutes, or until firm but still pliable. Chimichurri drizzled over the top.

19.Recipe for Seared Scallops with White Beans and Spinach

You'll need two strips of bacon, cut into small pieces. You can eat the bacon whole, but it only has about 18 calories per serving and adds a lot of flavor to the dish.

12 red onions, 1 clove of garlic, and 1 can (14 ounces) of rinsed and drained white beans (there are

many different kinds of white beans sold in cans). Cannellini beans are the best choice, but any will do.)

4 cups baby spinach 1 pound of large sea scallops Salt and black pepper to taste 1 tablespoon butter 1 lemon juice HOW TO MAKE IT

The bacon should be cooked until it begins to crisp.

Include the garlic and onion; 2 to 3 minutes, or until the onion is translucent and soft, sauté.

Simmer the spinach and beans until the spinach is wilted and the beans are hot. Stay warm.

Set a large saute pan or cast-iron skillet to medium-high heat.

Salt and pepper the scallops on both sides after blotting them dry with a paper towel.

Sear the scallops in the pan with the butter for 2 to 3 minutes on each side, until they are deeply caramelized.

Add the lemon juice to the beans just before serving. Add salt and pepper to taste.

Place scallops on top of the beans and divide them among four warm bowls or plates.

20.Quick Teriyaki Scallops Wrapped in Bacon Recipe

Eight large sea scallops are required. If at all possible, purchase "dry" scallops, which are wild and natural. "Wet" scallops have been soaked in a solution of a preservative, which lowers their quality and raises their cost due to their increased weight.)

4 to 8 strips of bacon marinated in teriyaki sauce (thin bacon works best here because it crisps up faster and prevents your scallops from overcooking). How to Make It: Marinate the scallops in enough teriyaki sauce to cover them, in the refrigerator, for 30 minutes.

Set the broiler to high. Wrap each scallop in just enough bacon to cover it completely without overlapping (the best way to crisp up the bacon is to stretch it thinly).

To secure, insert a toothpick through the bacon and scallop. Place in the oven six inches below the broiler and brush with a little more of the teriyaki marinade.

Cook for 10 to 12 minutes, or until the bacon is cooked through and the scallops are firm.

21. A Delectable Miso-Glazed Scallops Recipe
WHAT YOU NEED: 12 cups white miso paste, 12 cups sake, 14 cups sugar, and 14 cups canola oil. 1 lb large scallops, tough membranes removed. 2 cups

sugar snap peas. 12 tablespoons sesame oil. Salt and black pepper to taste. HOW TO MAKE IT: Whisk together the miso, sake, sugar, and oil in a mixing bowl.

Cover a small bowl with one-fourth of the mixture, refrigerate, and serve. Turn the scallops over in the remaining miso and marinate for up to 12 hours in the refrigerator.

Set the broiler to high.

A large cast-iron skillet or oiled baking sheet should be placed six inches below the broiler.

Pat the scallops dry after removing them from the marinade.

Sesame oil, salt, and pepper to taste, and toss the sugar snaps together.

Remove the sugar snaps and scallops with care and arrange them on the baking sheet when the sheet is very hot.

Broil for 5 to 6 minutes, or until the sugar snaps are tender and the scallops are thoroughly browned and firm.

With a drizzle of the miso sauce that was left over, serve the snap peas and scallops.

22. The Best Recipe for Classic Linguine with Clams

You will need four strips of bacon, cut into thin strips; one red onion, diced; two cloves of garlic, minced; a generous pinch of red pepper flakes; 32 cleaned littleneck clams; one cup dry white wine; twelve ounces of whole wheat linguine; one-fourth cup fresh chopped parsley leaves. Flat-leaf parsley, also known as Italian parsley, is a great and versatile herb that can be used to garnish pasta, soups, and soft scram

HOW TO MAKE IT Place the bacon in a large sauté pan or skillet over medium heat. In about 5 minutes, cook until the bacon is well browned and the fat renders.

Reserve the bacon after removing it; eliminate all but a very thin layer of the fat.

Add the onion, garlic, and pepper flakes to the heated pan.

Cook the onion for about three minutes, stirring occasionally, until it becomes translucent.

Continue to cook the clams and wine over medium heat until most of the wine has evaporated and the clams have opened, about 10 minutes. Cover the pan with a lid if the clams aren't opening. Any that never open, throw out.)

The pasta should be cooked according to the package until it is tender but still al dente.

Add the cooked linguine directly to the pan with the clams after draining the pasta and reserving about a cup of the cooking water.

Add a little pasta water if the noodles appear dry, and stir in the parsley after 30 seconds. 23.Lighter Clam Chowder Recipe: 4 strips chopped bacon, 1 small onion diced, 2 ribs diced celery, 1 tablespoon flour, 1 can (6.5 oz) drained clams, reserved juices, 2 cups clam juice, 1 cup milk, 2 medium Yukon gold potatoes peeled and diced (about 1 12 cups), 2 branches fresh thyme (optional), salt and black pepper to taste HOW TO MAKE IT: Cook the bacon in

Reserve on a plate lined with paper towels.

Cook for about five minutes, until the onions and celery are soft, in the bacon fat.

To get rid of the taste of raw flour, stir in the flour and cook for one minute.

Pour in the milk, the bottled clam juice, and the reserved clam juices, stirring constantly to incorporate the flour evenly.

Add the potatoes and, if using, the thyme to the simmering mixture. Cook the potatoes for about 10 minutes, or just until they are tender.

Add salt and black pepper to taste.

Add the clams just before serving and simmer until heated through.

Sprinkle the remaining bacon on top.

23.Grilled Mahi Mahi with Salsa Verde

YOU'LL NEED: 4 cups chopped fresh parsley, 4 cups chopped fresh mint (optional), 1 lemon juice, 4 cups olive oil, plus more for grilling, 2 to 3 anchovy fillets, minced, 2 tablespoons capers, rinsed, and chopped, 2 cloves garlic, finely minced, pinch of red pepper flakes, salt, and black pepper to taste, 4 mahi mahi fillets Make sure to clean and oil the grate.

In a mixing bowl, combine the parsley, mint, lemon juice, olive oil, anchovies, capers, garlic, and pepper flakes.

Add black pepper to taste.

Put the verde salsa aside.

After coating the fish in a thin layer of oil, sprinkle it with salt and pepper all over.

If you mess with the fish before it is ready to flip, it is likely to stick. Place the fillets on the grill, skin side down, and grill for 5 minutes, or until the skin is lightly charred, crisp, and pulls away easily.

Cook the other side for another 2 to 3 minutes, or until the fish flakes easily with your fingertip.

Spoon the salsa verde over the fillets as you serve them.

24.A Spicy Grilled Mahi-Mahi with Red Pepper Sauce

You'll Need: 1 jar (12 oz) roasted red peppers that have been drained; 12 teaspoons cayenne pepper; 1 clove garlic; 2 tablespoons olive oil; 1 tablespoon sherry or red wine vinegar; 12 teaspoons ground cumin; salt and black pepper to taste; 4 fillets of mahi-mahi, sea bass, halibut, or snapper (6 Add salt and pepper to taste. This sauce isn't just for fish. On grilled steak, pork chops, roasted chicken, or tossed with grilled vegetables, it is delicious.)

Heat a grill pan or stovetop grill pan with a little oil until medium-hot. Salt and pepper lightly the flesh side of the fillets before placing them, skin side down, on the hot grill.

Until the skins are lightly charred and crispy, cook for 4 to 5 minutes.

Cook for another two to three minutes on the other side.

When they're done, gently press on the fish with your fingertip to break it up.

With a heaping scoop of harissa, serve right away.

25.Honey-Mustard Glazed Salmon with Roasted Asparagus Recipe

4 salmon fillets (6 ounces each) Roasted Parmesan Asparagus Recipe: 1 tbsp butter, 1 tbsp brown sugar, 2 tbsp Dijon mustard, 1 tbsp honey, 1 tbsp soy sauce, 12 tbsp olive oil, salt and black pepper to taste In a microwave-safe bowl, combine the brown sugar and butter and microwave for 30 seconds to melt together.

Add the honey, mustard, and soy sauce by stirring.

In an oven-safe skillet, heat the oil to a high temperature.

Add the salmon, flesh side down, to the pan and season it with salt and pepper.

Flip after 3 to 4 minutes of cooking time until fully browned.

Place the pan in the oven and brush with half of the glaze. Bake for about 5 minutes, or until the salmon is firm and flaky but no white fat has formed on the surface.

Take the salmon out, brush it with more honey mustard, and serve it with the asparagus.

26. Sweet Chili-Glazed Salmon

You'll Need: 4 salmon fillets, 4–6 ounces each; 14 cup Asian-style sweet chilli sauce; 2 tablespoons of low-sodium soy sauce; 1 tablespoon grated fresh ginger; 1 teaspoon sriracha or another spicy chilli sauce. Despite its higher price, it contains fewer PCBs, toxins, and mercury than the majority of farmed varieties. Additionally, it tastes better.)

Preheat the oven to 425°F. HOW TO MAKE IT

In a bowl, combine the ginger, sriracha, soy sauce, and sweet chilli sauce.

Place the salmon fillets on a baking sheet lined with foil. Apply the chilli glaze to the salmon with a brush or a spoon.

Depending on the thickness of the fish, bake the salmon for approximately 10 minutes or until the glaze has begun to lightly caramelise and the salmon flakes easily with gentle pressure.

27. Recipe for Healthy Scrambled Eggs with Salmon, Asparagus, and Goat Cheese

You'll Need: 1 tablespoon butter 8 stalks of asparagus (with the woody bottoms removed), chopped into 1" pieces Salt and black pepper to taste 8 eggs (Spend an extra dollar or two on the highest-quality eggs you can find). The best eggs come from farmers markets where they are free to roam.)

2 tablespoons fat-free milk, 1 cup crumbled fresh goat cheese, and 4 ounces chopped smoked salmon.
HOW TO MAKE IT:
Heat the butter in a large sauté pan or nonstick skillet over medium heat.

Add the asparagus and cook until just tender (or "crisp-tender" in kitchen parlance) when the butter starts to foam. Add salt and pepper to taste.

Whisk the milk and the eggs together in a large bowl.

Add some salt and pepper to taste and to the pan with the asparagus.

Use a wooden spoon to constantly stir and scrape the eggs until they begin to form soft curds. Reduce the heat to low. Stir in the goat cheese one minute before they are finished.

When the eggs are still creamy and soft, remove them from the heat and fold in the smoked salmon. Keep in mind that scrambled eggs, like meat, continue to cook even after the heat is turned off.

28.A Quick and Easiest Roast Salmon with Lentils Recipe

WHAT YOU NEED: 12 tablespoons olive oil; one medium carrot that has been peeled and diced; one medium yellow onion that has been diced; two cloves of minced garlic; one cup of dried lentils; three cups of chicken broth or water; two bay leaves; two tablespoons of red wine vinegar; salt and black pepper to taste; four salmon fillets that weigh four ounces each; two tablespoons of Dijon mustard

In a medium saucepan, heat the olive oil to a medium temperature.

Sauté the carrot, onion, and garlic for 5 to 7 minutes, or until lightly browned and soft.

Lentils, broth, and bay leaves should be added.

Cook the lentils for about 20 minutes, or until they are tender and most of the liquid has evaporated.

Add the vinegar, season with salt and pepper, and remove the bay leaves before serving.

Roast the salmon while the lentils simmer: Add salt and black pepper to the fish.

Spread the mustard and brown sugar evenly over the salmon fillets in a mixing bowl.

The salmon should be placed on a baking sheet and baked on the highest oven rack. Roast the salmon for 8 to 10 minutes, or until it flakes easily with your finger's gentle pressure and the surface is browned.

Divide the lentils among four plates or pasta bowls and add a piece of salmon to the top of each serving.

29. The Best Grilled Salmon with Ginger Soy Butter

You'll Need: 2 tablespoons softened unsalted butter; 2 tablespoons minced chives; 2 tablespoons grated fresh ginger; 1 lemon juice; 2 tablespoons low-sodium soy sauce; 4 salmon fillets (4–6 ounces each); salt and black pepper to taste; 1 tablespoon olive oil. Place aside.

Prepare a grill or grill pan for use.

Rub the oil into the salmon after seasoning it with salt and pepper.

Rub the grill grates with an oil-soaked paper towel after cleaning them.

Cook the salmon, skin side down, for 4 to 5 minutes, or until the skin is crisp and lightly charred.

Cook the fish over on the flesh side for another 2 to 3 minutes, or until the flesh flakes easily with your finger but is still slightly translucent in the middle. We recommend serving salmon medium-rare, but if you want it fully cooked, leave it on for another two to three minutes.)

A generous spoonful of the flavoured butter, which should begin to melt upon contact, should be served alongside the salmon.

Chapter five
Poultry and meat mains

1. Lean proteins like chicken are important first foods for infants and toddlers (0 to 2 years old) because they contain iron, zinc, protein, choline, and long chain polyunsaturated fatty acids. Choline chicken also contains vitamins and minerals that help the brain function. Chicken contains choline, a nutrient that is essential for a child's normal brain development but is lacking in pregnant or lactating women. In point of fact, choline contributes to overall health across the lifespan. Choline is essential for brain development in young children, and recent studies have even shed light on its role in influencing mood and maintaining cognitive function into adulthood.

2. High-Quality Protein Chicken Strengthens Muscles A roasted, boneless, and skinless 3.5-ounce chicken breast contains approximately 31 grams of protein. However, in comparison to many plant-based proteins, the protein from chicken stands out because it is of a higher quality and contains sufficient amounts of each of the nine essential amino acids—the building blocks of protein—that humans require in their diet. The nine essential amino acids can only be obtained from food, and many plant-derived foods have a less favorable amino acid profile, making them less digestible and less useful to the body.

3. Why Choose Chicken? Dark-meat chicken cuts are packed with nutrients.

In comparison to white meat cuts, dark meat typically contains more vitamins and minerals, such as iron and zinc, as well as riboflavin, thiamin, and vitamins B6 and B12. Due to its juicy, tender texture, dark meat also has more flavor and is less likely to dry out or become overly chewy during cooking. Here is a cut-by-cut nutritional comparison of dark meat versus white meat chicken. Chicken with white or dark meat is nutritious and can be included in a healthy diet.

4. Healthy fats like unsaturated fats can be substituted for unhealthy fats like saturated fats and trans fats in a diet to improve heart health. Unsaturated fats Unsaturated fats Chicken Helps Heart Health Although chicken does provide unsaturated fat, red meat generally contains more saturated (bad) fat than chicken. Chicken is also America's favorite high-quality, low-fat, low-sodium, and low-cholesterol source of protein. It is one of the top two heart-healthy diets, and many studies show that eating lean chicken reduces your risk of heart disease. In point of fact, a recent study involving over 1.4 million people who were followed for 30 years found no connection between eating poultry, including chicken. The lack of a link between lean poultry and heart disease, according to the researchers, may be attributable to its low saturated fat content.

5. Vitamin B12: Chicken is good for our brains. Chicken contains tryptophan, an amino acid linked to rising levels of the neurochemical serotonin, also known as the "feel good" chemical. It contains vitamin B12 and choline, which together, may advance mental health in kids, help the sensory system capability appropriately and help mental execution in more established grown-ups.

Vitamin B12 is a nutrient that helps make your body's DNA and keeps nerve and blood cells healthy! Vitamin B12, which is found in both dark and white meat chicken, may assist in the proper functioning of the nervous system, improve cognitive performance in older adults, and promote brain development in children. Skinless dark meat chicken thigh weighs 3.5 ounces and provides 0.42 micrograms of vitamin B12, which is the recommended daily intake.

There you have it, then! Five chicken health benefits you didn't know about! Are you looking for ideas for recipes that will put your newfound knowledge to the test in tasty, original, and simple ways? Chicken Roost has these delicious recipes!

Chapter six
Best snacks
and sweet treat

1. Mixed nuts are an excellent source of healthy fats, protein, and fiber, making them an ideal snack.

They are very filling, have a lot of health benefits, and are delicious. Additionally, despite their higher calorie and fat content, nuts may help you lose weight when consumed in moderation, according to studies.

Walnuts, almonds, Brazil nuts, hazelnuts, pine nuts, macadamia nuts, cashews, and pistachios are just a few of the many types of nuts available.

They are a great option for on-the-go snacking because they do not require refrigeration. Keep your portion sizes to about 1 ounce, or 1/4 cup, at all times.

2. Guacamole and red bell pepper The combination of guacamole and red bell peppers gives you a lot of nutrients that help you feel full for hours.

Even though all bell peppers are good for you, the red ones have a lot of antioxidants. On the other hand, guacamole is a good source of fiber, vitamins A, B, and C, healthy fats, and minerals like potassium and phosphorus.

The combination of one large red bell pepper and three ounces (85 grams) of guacamole gives this snack the best of both worlds while keeping its calorie count below 200

3. Greek yogurt, mixed berries, and plain Greek yogurt make a tasty, nutrient-dense snack.

Greek yogurt has a lot of protein, and berries are one of the best sources of antioxidants. Add a variety of different colored berries to your yoghourt to get a variety of nutrients and a sweet and sour taste.

4. Slices of apple with peanut butter Marie delle Donne/Offset Images Peanut butter and apples are a nutritional and flavor match made in heaven.

Apples are, on the one hand, a fruit high in fiber. On the other hand, peanuts contain healthy fats, plant-based protein, and fiber, which are basically all of the filling nutrients you should look for in a snack. If you combine apples with peanut butter, you can have a snack that is both crisp and creamy. For a boost in flavor, sprinkle some cinnamon on top.

Keep in mind that numerous brands of store-bought peanut butter contain oil and sugar additions. Choose one that only has salt and peanuts on the ingredient list.

5. Fruit and cottage cheese Cottage cheese has 24 grams of protein per cup, making it a filling snack. When you combine the fiber in the fruit with the protein and fat in the cheese, you get a sweet, creamy, and filling snack.

When paired with tropical fruits like pineapple, papaya, or watermelon, the combination is exceptional.

6. Celery sticks with cream cheese are a traditional low-carb snack that can help you feel full for longer.

You'll be able to enjoy a snack packed with fiber that combines the crunch of the celery with the creaminess of the cheese. Another crunchy and creamy combination is celery sticks and peanut butter or almond butter.

A serving of five small celery sticks and 30 grams of cream cheese has approximately 100 calories. Chips made of kale Kale is a great source of minerals like calcium and phosphorus, as well as fiber and antioxidants like beta carotene, lutein, and zeaxanthin. Kale has a lower concentration of oxalic acid, an antinutrient that prevents calcium from being absorbed, than many other leafy greens. When paired with olive oil, kale produces crispier chips that are also more nutritious and filling.

About 150 calories are provided by this simple recipe for kale chips:

Kale chips contain:

Ingredients: 1 cup (20 grams) of chopped kale leaves; 1 tablespoon (15 milliliters) of olive oil; 1/4 teaspoon (1.5 grams) of salt.

In a bowl, combine all ingredients. Bake the kale for 10 to 15 minutes at 350°F (175°C) on a baking sheet lined with parchment until crispy and beginning to slightly brown. They can easily burn, so keep an eye on them.

7.Ingredients for chia seed pudding

1 tablespoon (15 grams) of chia seeds, 1/3 cup (80 mL) of your preferred dairy or non-dairy milk, 1/2 teaspoon (8 grams) of cocoa powder or peanut butter for flavor, 1/2 cup (75 grams) of mixed berries, 1–2 teaspoons of sweetener, such as honey or maple syrup, if desired Instructions:

In a small bowl or jar, combine the chia seeds and the liquid of your choice. Refrigerate the jar for at least 30 minutes with a cover. Add peanut butter or cocoa powder and sweetener. Add the berries on top.

8. Beets It has been discovered that the natural nitrates in beets increase blood flow throughout the body, particularly to the brain, thereby enhancing focus and concentration.

Try Sweet & Beets from Terra Chips for a quick and easy snack to keep on hand at work. They are a delicious combination of sweet potatoes and beets that your entire workplace will enjoy.

9.Rosemary According to a recent study, just the smell of rosemary can lead to improved memory. One of rosemary oil's main chemicals, 1,8-cineole, has been shown to improve brain performance. In a recent study, higher levels of 1,8-cineole were associated with improved test speed and accuracy.

10.Chocolate Strawberry Chia Pudding
Ingredients: 1 cup (250 mL) chocolate milk; 14 cup (60 mL) chia seeds; 4 quartered strawberries. SPECIAL EQUIPMENT: Two 8-ounce glass jars with lids. Instructions: Pour 12 cups (250 mL) of chocolate milk into each jar. Each jar should have three tbsp (30 mL) of the chia seeds added, and stir to combine.

Equally divide the strawberries among the jars.
Refrigerate each jar for the night with a cover.

11.Balls or bites
These bite-sized, portion-controlled snacks can
quickly quell sweet cravings. You can meal plan for
the week and make a few healthy energy balls or
bites. Numerous recipes incorporate chocolate,
coconuts, nuts, seeds, and dried fruit like dates. To
get you started, here is a delicious recipe for Peanut
Butter Banana Energy Bites. You can also buy
ready-made energy balls or bites at some coffee
shops.

12. Making homemade trail mix can be done in
less than five minutes, and it can help those who
enjoy both sweet and savory foods at the same time.
Combine one cup of unsalted roasted nuts, such as
cashews, pistachios, or almonds, to make a healthy,
sweet trail mix; one cup of dried fruit, such as
mangoes, tart cherries, cranberries, raisins, or
apricots; and dark chocolate chips, quarter cup.
Divide into quarter-cup portions and toss together.
Divide the food into individual portions to reduce
calories and make it simple to grab and go from the
pantry.

Chapter seven
Dressing and sauce

1. Try dairy products with fewer calories. Many sauces and dressings that have a lot of calories and fat are made with cream. Some of these smooth and creamy sauces can really add calories if you use heavy cream, full-fat buttermilk, or sour cream.[2] However, keep in mind that some companies make up for the lack of fat by adding extra salt or sugar.

The flavor of many dressings and sauces comes from dairy products that are higher in calories and fat. The fact that these ingredients contain more calories is a drawback.

It can be difficult to completely eliminate dairy, so use dairy products with fewer calories to reduce your overall fat and calorie intake.

For instance, you can utilize without fat harsh cream to make dressings or utilize low-fat buttermilk to make farm dressing.

2. Substitute cream-based sauces for nuts. You might be surprised to learn that nuts can be used to make traditionally higher-calorie dairy dressings and sauces[3]. This is a great way to boost the nutrition of some of your favorite sauces.

Some of those sauces with more calories can be made better by adding nuts. Minerals, protein, and healthy fats are all abundant in nuts.

Nuts have a lot of calories, but they also have a lot of protein, good fats, and minerals that traditional sauces made with cream don't have.

Nuts also have a lot of fat, but the kind of fat in them that is good for your heart is called omega-3 fat. It has been demonstrated that this kind of fat is good for your heart.[4] To use nuts as the base of creamy sauces, you need to soak them in hot water to make them soft. After that, combine them with your preferred seasonings and blend or puree them.

3. Trim excess fat. Getting rid of the actual fat in seasonings and sauces is another way to cut back on calories and fat.

Because the fat from the meat cannot be removed or strained, some sauces, like meat sauce, can contain a lot of fat.

For instance, after browning the meat for bolognese sauce, drain the excess fat. Alternately, you can skim off the fat from the top of the sauce by letting it cool in the refrigerator, which helps the fat solidify.

4. Reduce the amount of salt. Many dressings and sauces have more problems than just fat and calories as a whole. The amount of salt or sodium can also be a problem.

Consuming too much sodium or salt may raise your risk of high blood pressure, which in turn raises your risk of stroke.

Start by limiting the amount of salt you actually add to your sauce or dressing when making your own homemade sauces. Also, make sure you always measure the salt you use.[5] You could also use other ingredients to give your sauce or dressing that kick of flavor that comes from salt. Vinegar, a hot pepper, or lemon juice are some examples. Spices like ginger, garlic, dried herbs, and others can also enhance flavor.

5. Make use of natural components to imitate flavors. Try using natural ingredients like fruits and vegetables if you want to sweeten a sauce or add more flavor. Without adding a lot of calories or fat, these can add a lot of flavor.

Naturally low in calories, fruits and vegetables are rich in vitamins and fiber. They also have a lot of great flavor that can be used in dressings and sauces. Try pureeing fruit, for instance, if you want to make a sweet sauce or add a little sweetness to something.

In addition, you can incorporate roasted vegetables like roasted red peppers for a touch of smoky sweetness into dressings and sauces.

6. Make blue cheese dressing that is healthier. Enjoy this low-calorie version of the creamy classic dressing. Mash up about 1/2 cup of crumbled blue cheese and 6 ounces of plain fat-free Greek yoghourt in a small bowl to maintain the creaminess.[6]Mix about 1/2 cup of crumbled blue cheese and 6 ounces of plain fat-free Greek yogurt in a small bowl. It is not necessary for the blue cheese to be completely smooth; it can instead be as chunky or smooth as you like.

The blue cheese mixture should have one tablespoon each of white wine vinegar, lemon juice, and mayonnaise. Also add a pinch of garlic powder and stir.

Adjust the amount of salt and pepper to taste in your dressing. Serve over your favorite salad after chilling for at least 30 minutes.

7. Mix a vegan Alfredo sauce together. This vegan Alfredo sauce made from nuts is perfect for Alfredo lovers. The only dairy in this recipe is pureed nuts, which give it a wonderful creamy texture[7]. To begin, soak half a cup of raw cashews in water for a good amount of time. If possible, allow them to soak for at least eight hours.

In addition to the cashews that have been soaked, add 1 teaspoon of garlic to a blender. Puree the vegetables with about 3/4 cup of vegetable broth until almost smooth.

Add salt and pepper to taste, as well as 1/4 cup nutritional yeast (or more or less, depending on your preferences) and 1 tablespoon (14.8 milliliters) of lemon juice.

Blend once more until smooth. Season with salt and pepper as needed. Additionally, if the sauce is too thick, add some additional broth.

Serve with some extra nutritional yeast and chopped basil served over your favorite pasta.

8. Make a cheese sauce with fewer calories. A cheese sauce is the only thing that can make plain steamed broccoli or cauliflower taste better. This delicious recipe is low in calories.[8] Whisk 5 tablespoons (73.9 milliliters) of flour with 1/4 cup low-fat milk until smooth in a small bowl.

In a sauce pan, combine the flour mixture with another 1 cup of milk and heat on medium-high until it just begins to simmer.

To keep the milk mixture from burning or becoming clumpy, constantly whisk it. It will need about four minutes to cook until it becomes thick.

Stir in 1/3 cup shredded cheddar, 1 teaspoon dry mustard, 1/2 teaspoon paprika, and salt and pepper to taste after removing from heat.

Your cheese sauce can be drizzled on blanched vegetables or homemade nachos.

9. Try spices and herbs. Even though dressings and sauces can enhance the flavor of many dishes, there are still ways to flavor foods without adding any calories.

Foods can benefit from the flavor of dried or fresh herbs and spices without the calories or fat.

You can learn to enjoy foods with minimal added sauces or dressings by adding fresh herbs to a tomato-based pasta sauce or rubbing a steak with a flavorful spice blend.

10. Employ seasonal produce. If they aren't in season or fresh, some foods may taste a little bland. You might want to add a dressing or sauce to boost their flavor because of this. You can cut down on the amount of flavoring you need by using things that are in season.

There will be a selection of seasonal fruits and vegetables at any given time. Blackberries and strawberries, for instance, are in season during the summer. In the fall and winter, butternut squash and kale are in season.

When you use fresh ingredients, their flavor is more pronounced and vibrant. You might not need to add a dressing or sauce with a lot of calories to make them taste better.

11. Try cooking with a lot of flavor. Some cooking techniques give foods a lot of flavor, while others make them taste a little bland. Try using cooking methods that can help your food taste better.

Steaming, for example, imparts little flavor to foods when cooked. Consequently, drizzlingThat's why it's so appealing to drizzle cheese sauce over just steamed broccoli.

Foods that are steamed, sautéed, boiled, or poached don't always have a lot of flavor. Skip these cooking methods in favor of something a little more flavorful to help you get used to using less of those sauces and dressings with more calories.

Grilling is a great way to cook that is also healthy and gives foods a lot of flavor. Foods like proteins, vegetables, and even fruits get a great sear on the outside when they are grilled. Without adding any dressings, this gives flavors a great smoky, charred flavor.[10] Roasting is another great method, especially for vegetables. The process of roasting involves slowly caramelizing and browning foods on the outside using the oven's high temperature. They soften, get nutty, and become sweet. Sauces and dressings are not required here either.

12. Use dressings and sauces with more calories in moderation. Even though there are a lot of low-calorie recipes and ways to add more flavor to foods, you can still use your favorite dressings and sauces from time to time.

It is usually not recommended to use a sauce with more calories or fat frequently. Even in smaller amounts, these can increase your daily calorie intake.

You can still include some of your favorite foods if you use them in moderation and portion out the right amount. Instead of pouring dressings or sauces over your dish or mixing them in, try dipping foods in them. When dipping, most people use less dressing.

The serving size can be found on the nutrition label. Serving sizes for dressings and sauces typically range from one to two tablespoons. You will need to take into account the additional fat and calories if you use more.

Also, be careful with the low-fat or fat-free products you buy at the store. While the amount of sodium and/or sugar is often higher, the fat content is frequently lower. Additionally, the reduced total calories rarely outweigh the additional ingredients.

The best option is to prepare a healthier version at home to use most of the time and occasionally indulge in moderation in the "real deal."

Made in the USA
Monee, IL
14 September 2023

42742234R00090